the triggering event

The true key to long-term weight loss

Beth Duffus

ISBN: 978-1-326-11397-1

PublishNation, London
www.publishnation.co.uk

Contents

Acknowledgements

Thanks to Anne Stark and Jacqueline Collins for proof-reading, feedback and much appreciated moral support.

Introduction

I write this at a time when there are more than twice the number of people who are overweight or obese on the planet than those who are threatened with starvation: 2 billion to 840 million respectively.[1,2] It is a chilling statistic that represents a rising public health emergency that stretches across the world. The speed with which this has escalated in the last fifty years, especially the last twenty, is unprecedented. In the UK alone, around 60% of the adult population over the age of 16 are overweight, including 26% who are clinically obese, and childhood obesity remains worryingly high.[3] It is getting worse. Current trends predict that by 2050 between 50-60% of UK adults will be clinically obese – our children's generation.[4]

The sharp rise in the prevalence of excess weight and obesity in recent decades cannot be explained by evolution; it takes hundreds of generations for evolutionary change to take place. One theory that is gaining traction suggests that a significant proportion of the population, perhaps as much as 50-60%, is genetically predisposed to gain weight, given the right circumstances. This is the so-called 'hungry gene'.[5] In evolutionary terms, this would have conferred a considerable advantage: the ability to fatten up in times of plenty, so that you have your own personal fuel tank in times of scarcity. Paradoxically, in today's fast-food, sedentary environment, this predisposition poses a threat to health, and it is proving to be a tough problem to throw into reverse.

The World Health Organisation, the worldwide scientific community and government organisations are trying to address the root causes of this obesity pandemic. It is generally accepted, however, that it may take decades to correct, and there are substantial obstacles. It is not just the implications for physical health, or social and medical costs that give cause for concern, serious as these are. Being significantly overweight or obese also causes great unhappiness and despair, especially for those who feel it prevents them from living life to the full.

I have been a UK registered nurse for almost 30 years, and I have an academic background in philosophy. I have worked in a wide range of hospital and community settings often supporting patients with chronic conditions associated with poor lifestyle choices. Being overweight or obese is an especially complex problem, however, and the stock advice – to just eat less and move more – has a poor track record. This advice exasperates patients and leaves healthcare professionals feeling demoralised, so I am under no illusion about how difficult a problem this is. Ineffective mainstream advice, impenetrable academic research and dry government reports leave the overweight individual on the ground a bit stranded. So, I decided to take a more in-depth look at what was really on offer for people who wanted to lose weight, and to find out why so many seemed to fail.

I discovered that people who are overweight or obese are trapped in a triangle of competing forces. On one side is a list of health risks associated with being overweight; on another is seductively marketed food that is cheap, abundant and palatable; on the third side is the lucrative dieting and fitness industry that sells a steady stream of quick-fix promises that rarely deliver. This triangle ties anyone struggling with their weight into an endless loop of anxiety, false hope, failing willpower and guilt. I realised that long-term success in reaching and sustaining a healthy weight depends on breaking out of this triangle for good. I look at these factors in more detail in the next chapter because it is important to understand the way in which we are manipulated into accepting certain beliefs and associations by the advertising industry, social pressures and life experience.

The beliefs we hold are the very levers of our lives. Many of our beliefs have been carried throughout life from childhood and are so embedded in our thinking we mistake them for truths. We can be so immersed in them that we can no longer see them clearly, or how they steer our lives. Beliefs dictate our thoughts, feelings and actions; they have considerable influence on the outcomes of our lives. But if we are able to identify the beliefs that prevent us from living life the way we want to, we can challenge and transform them into something far more constructive.

For example, it is generally believed that it is difficult to maintain significant weight loss in the long-term. A failure rate as high as 95% is often quoted in the press, though I have been unable to track down any reliable evidence which supports this figure. The self-confidence needed to lose weight is likely to be undermined by such a colossal failure rate. But what if it is wrong? What if the success rate for long-term weight loss is actually much higher, under the right circumstances? Surely knowing this would create a sense of optimism and resolve on the journey towards a normal, healthy weight?

I decided to track down as much information as possible about people who had maintained substantial weight loss over time to see what distinguished them from those who repeatedly failed to do so. In addition to research studies and books which focus on this group, it was helpful to find the National Weight Control Registry (NWCR), which is run by a research team at the University of Colorado in the USA. The NWCR team do not run any weight-loss programmes, but they maintain a register of adults who have lost 30 lbs or more and sustained this for over a year. In fact, most members have lost far more weight than this, and kept it off for several years, even decades. At the time of writing there are over 10,000 people registered with the NWCR.

Many studies have been carried out with this group, but they tend to focus on which diets were followed and how much exercise was taken. This does not really distinguish the members of this group from the legions of dieters who fail to achieve long-term weight loss using the same methods. As I read through the studies and the case histories, however, one thing stood out: the trigger for permanent change was a sudden moment or event that transformed beliefs and behaviours. It was quite different from anything experienced before. These events may or may not seem dramatic to the outside observer, but to the individual they were extraordinary and they had an immediate impact. Lifestyles were amended at once, and the journey to a normal weight and health was undertaken for the final time. This is what really separates those who successfully maintain weight loss from those who do not. It supports my theory about the central role that beliefs play in our lives, and it is worth exploring in more depth.

These triggering events take many forms. Some people had a health scare, or had a relative die from an obesity-related illness. Others reached an all-time high weight, or realised how much money they had squandered on diet products over the years. Some saw the extent to which their lives were being ruled by diets, or how they had become defined by being overweight. The list is long and highly personal; what works for one person may not for another. Significantly, nearly all those who managed to sustain weight loss for long periods had tried and failed to do so many times before. The final, successful attempt was marked by a shift in attitude brought on by a triggering event.

But what does someone do if they have had no such triggering event, or at least not one powerful enough to effect permanent change? It is clearly too extreme to wait for a health crisis. Is there a way to intentionally create the same effect; one that would have the same powerful impact on thinking and behaviour? I sincerely believe that there is, but it is no simple matter. Even identifying the deep-seated beliefs we hold in the first place is a tall order, and requires much self-reflection. It is a very personal journey, but one that must be taken if someone is to understand why they act as they do. Only then can the process of challenging beliefs and replacing them with ones that are more liberating and life-enhancing begin.

Although the main focus of this book is exploring the role that beliefs have in our lives, particularly with regard to health and weight, I am also concerned about our culture of dieting. Veteran dieters will be familiar with the weight-loss diets that are currently fashionable. They range from low-carbohydrate diets to low-fat diets to intermittent fasting regimes, all with their own devoted supporters. Then there are more extreme diets, for example those that involve drinking nothing but vegetable juice, or eating only raw food. Several of these diets promise rapid weight loss, which, I believe, exploits the despair experienced by those who are overweight. A significant body of evidence shows that rapid weight loss causes rebound weight gain, and is a fast-track to obesity. I decided, therefore, to include a chapter on the detrimental effects of rapid weight-loss diets, in the hope of persuading people to steer well clear of them.

Trapped in the Triangle

As I explored the obesity and weight loss scene, three strong themes emerged: the relentless quest for slimness pushed by the dieting and fitness industry; the abundance of fattening food and drink within our society; and significant health risks. They each exert a powerful psychological force, and they compete with and contradict one another. I saw that anyone who is overweight or obese is trapped by these opposing influences. They seem to be stuck within a triangle which bounces them between false promises, fear, guilt and recrimination. But I also saw that this trap is an illusion of wrong beliefs created by life experience, aggressive marketing techniques and scare tactics from those in perceived positions of authority. Breaking out of this trap necessarily means questioning those beliefs but first it is worth considering how they thrive within our society in the first place.

THE DIETING INDUSTRY

Although I knew the dieting industry was big business, I did not know the territory was quite so vast. On Amazon's UK website alone there are over 11,000 paperback books listed under 'losing weight', with hundreds more added each month. My investigations revealed a world of conflicting and inconsistent advice, only some of which is backed up by decent science. For example, a currently fashionable diet is based on shaky assumptions about the food eaten by prehistoric humans, another on even shakier beliefs about the need to 'detox' the body. A great deal of this advice is dispensed by people with no qualifications in healthcare, science or nutrition, though this does not seem to lessen their zeal. There is also not much evidence that the end results match the claims made by many of these weight-loss guides, either within the books themselves or from reviewers' comments.

Researching the customer reviews of a wide range of dieting books was a tiresome but revealing exercise. It gave me insight not just into the perceived pros and cons of a particular weight-loss book, but also into the mindset of the typical serial dieter. Often knowledgeable about the dieting industry, he or she constantly searches for answers and may express irritation if a book offers nothing new. There is early elation if weight has been lost and despair if it has not, but, as book reviews are typically posted within a few weeks of purchase, long-term success or failure goes unrecorded. It seemed to me that many dieters wanted to be told exactly what to do, as if there was some secret formula to being slim that they had missed somewhere along the line. I sensed that many reviewers had delegated responsibility for their weight loss to the authors of these books. When they failed to lose weight, the sense of betrayal was palpable, yet it was often qualified by self-chastisement, and a forlorn confession that instructions were not fully complied with. Nowhere, however, did I see anyone question the concept of these diets as the best route to long-term weight loss.

In addition to the huge number of dieting books, the range of slimming products also took me by surprise. Entire shelf units in high-street pharmacies are dedicated to them. They include many brand products that replace meals and snacks with milk shakes, soups or low calorie candy bars. There are also ranges of 'slimming aids', marketed to look like medicines, which claim to block carbohydrate absorption, or bind to dietary fat, or bulk up in the stomach to reduce the appetite. The active ingredients in some of these products cannot be disclosed, we are told, due to trademark protection, so consumers have no real idea what they are taking.

Unsurprisingly, all these slimming aids carry disclaimers stating that they must be used in conjunction with a balanced diet and exercise, so the manufacturers are off the hook if no weight loss ensues.

Experienced dieters will probably also be aware of the current vogue for capsules containing raspberry ketones, green coffee bean extract, acai berry or garcinia cambogia. Now, there is nothing to suggest that any of these substances are harmful if taken as instructed by the manufacturers, but at the time of writing there is also no good evidence to support the claim that they help much with weight loss either. Add to all this the wide range of pre-packaged food and drink products in supermarkets that are 'diet' or 'lite', or otherwise promoted as low-calorie or low-fat, and you start to see just how lucrative the dieting industry actually is.

As I became aware of just how many of these products are out there, and how aggressively they are promoted, I became quite angry. These products are expensive and the marketing techniques are exploitative. My heart went out to those who part with their hard-earned cash with an aching hope that this time they might have found the answer to their weight problem and the unhappiness it causes. Many will be disappointed when they discover they have not.

There is nothing new about the problem of being overweight or the desire to correct this. Our modern problem is a question of scale. Louise Foxcroft, in her book *Calories and Corsets: A history of dieting over 2,000 years,* gives an entertaining history of weight loss advice and the extent to which people desperate to slim down have always been vulnerable to crack-pot remedies.[6] Some of the adverts blinking at us from the internet suggests that not much has changed in this respect.

Interestingly, some of our forebears were not far off the right mark. As far back as the Middle Ages it was noticed that weight could be shed by avoiding bread and pastry. In the 18th century, expanding waistlines, and rotting teeth, were rightly connected to escalating sugar consumption in America and Europe. In 1860, the stout William Banting, who lived in London, rose to fame for his no-bread, no-potatoes, no-pastry, no-sugar diet. Banting, obese by today's standards, succeeded in losing weight for the first time in his life and published a letter outlining the regime, which is still available today.[7] Such was the popularity of his diet that it entered common parlance, and efforts to lose weight became known as 'banting' right into the early 20th century. Today we can recognise it as a low-carbohydrate diet.

Many of today's commentators would concur with Banting, but somewhere over the course of two world wars his message got lost. In the affluent post-war years, rates of heart disease and obesity rose in most Western countries, notably America. It was assumed that dietary fat was the cause because the coronary arteries of heart attack victims were found to be clogged with fatty plaques on post-mortem examination. It became accepted medical dogma that consuming too much fat, especially solidifying saturated fat, was a leading cause of cardiovascular disease. Anyone who challenged this was dismissed as a heretic. Low-fat diets were the acclaimed solution even though they were often dull and difficult to sustain. Many of these diets will still be familiar to today's generation of dieters. Slimming clubs appeared: Weight Watchers in the USA in 1963, and Slimming World in the UK in 1969. There were also brand-named diets such as The Scarsdale Diet, the F-Plan Diet and, later, the diet books of Rosemary Conley. These are just a few examples of thousands of low-fat diets and products that flooded onto the market. Many of these books continue to make good sales today.

It was the American doctor, Robert Atkins, who first put his head above the parapet in the 1970s by challenging the principles of the low-fat diet. By this time, rising trends in obesity were starting to cause concern in America and the UK. Atkins opposed mainstream medical opinion by arguing that it was the excessive consumption of carbohydrates that caused fatness and poor health, not dietary fat. Indeed, he argued that it was not at all harmful to consume unlimited amounts of protein and fat, including saturated fat.[8] The backlash from the medical establishment was forceful. Atkins was threatened with having his medical licence revoked on the grounds of giving negligent advice to patients, but he held his ground. It was difficult to deny that the Atkins Diet shifted the pounds off more rapidly than most low-fat diets. Significantly, there was also little evidence of rising levels of fat within the blood in those following his regime.[9] It has taken medical science forty years to concede that low-carbohydrate diets might be more effective than low-fat regimes for weight loss. It is now accepted that saturated fat is more benign that previously thought, but the argument about the link between dietary fat and cardiovascular disease rages on within the scientific community.

The dieting industry was quick to catch on. Literally thousands of low-carbohydrate dieting books are currently on the market. They come in many different guises, and it can be difficult to see at first that they are all saying essentially the same thing. Here is a small selection: the New Atkins Diet; the South Beach Diet; the Zone Diet; the Dolce Diet; the Dukan Diet; the diets of John Biffa; plus a long list of 'fitness trainer' or celebrity-endorsed diets. Not forgetting, of course, the high-selling range of 'paleo' diet books which tell us that all our weight problems will be solved if we simply return to the diet of our clean-living Palaeolithic ancestors. This has been a marketing coup if ever there was one, not least because it conveniently glosses over the fact that the lives of these early humans were so fragile and brutal that few lived past the age of thirty five.

The dieting scene is, of course, far more complex than a simple tension between just these two weight-loss strategies. There are also many books advocating low glycaemic index diets (based on so-called 'slow' carbohydrate foodstuffs), no-sugar diets, general low calorie diets, and more recently, intermittent fasting regimes.

Generally, these diets are safe and do-able, but there are so many options that it is little wonder that those wishing to lose weight become confused by it all. In spite of my cynicism about marketing tactics, none of the above are crank diets. I take issue with any diet that recommends one-off, rapid weight loss, however, and some versions of these diets do fall into that trap. I will return to this issue in a later chapter.

Needless to day, there are plenty of crank diets out there. I suggest that any diet promising rapid weigh-loss by consuming nothing but juiced vegetables, or nothing but raw fruit and vegetables, should be approached with caution. Even more extreme are the 'cleanser' diets based on water, lemon juice and cayenne pepper, or other similar very-low-calorie regimes. As reviewers' comments confirm, these diets can make some people feel weak and unwell, which is hardly surprising. Worryingly, some of these extreme diets target very young women with their choice of cover images, advertising strap lines and style of writing. And they sell!

It is worth pointing out that the whole concept of 'detoxing' the body is entirely bogus. The human body is a miracle of evolution and does a very excellent job of detoxing itself, particularly via the liver and kidneys. Anyone laying off alcohol and junk food for a few days is likely to feel better for it, but they should give credit to the natural, restorative mechanisms of their bodies, not some faddish and quite unnecessary 'detox' regime.

The psychological approach to weight loss is also a dominant theme within the dieting industry. This points to yet another division within the scientific community, which has argued for a long time about whether or not obesity is really a psychological problem, or even an eating disorder. Many dieters will be familiar with Paul McKenna's hypnotherapy books for weight loss, though he is by no means the only author in this genre. If book sales are anything to go by, he has been enormously successful with this approach, in addition to his books covering other topics such as self confidence and money. I believe that direct hypnotherapy can be quite useful, but it is highly individual and tricky to pull off as a one-size-fits-all book. If a book of this kind just happens to hit the right mark with a particular reader it might be quite effective, but, for many, it might not hit any mark at all.

The other psychological approach is to label overeating as emotional eating. I have never been convinced by this. I believe that bouts of excessive eating generally have one of two causes. Firstly, they may be linked to deeply held beliefs about deserving rewards or self-nurturing, bearing in mind that beliefs are not the same as emotions. Secondly, if weight has been lost rapidly after a period of strict dieting, the body will respond by generating a powerful physiological hunger that is almost impossible to resist. I call this 'deep hunger'. It is often the cause of episodes of binge eating and it is physical, not

12

emotional. Someone trying to lose weight is likely to have an emotional reaction to such overeating but this is effect, not cause. They may feel a sense of hopelessness or self-loathing if they mistakenly believe that the cause of their overeating is their lack of self-discipline, but it is the belief that is at fault, not the self-discipline. I return to both of these issues in the coming chapters.

THE FITNESS INDUSTRY

A new trend that emerged in the late 1960s was exercise for its own sake. Jogging, in particular, grew into a craze from the 1970s onwards. Those of us old enough to remember may have forgotten how odd it was to see people running in the streets in their gym kit, because today it is so commonplace. New style health clubs also emerged with cantilever weight machines, treadmills and stationary cycles. Previously, gyms had been sweaty places for boxers or body builders. Women were drawn in their thousands to aerobics classes and the new fashions for leotards, leggings and sweatbands. Expensive trainers became de rigueur and replaced the humble plimsoll. In the 1980s, many of us responded enthusiastically to Jane Fonda's call to 'feel the burn' to tone our muscles and lose as much body fat as possible. Her videos sold in millions and have been copied by a long list of celebrities and fitness trainers ever since. Many of us have at least one of these on our shelves.

Health club chains and franchises are now in almost every city the world. They maintain an atmosphere of exclusivity, and often double as social clubs with cafes or bars. 'Fitness trainers' carry out assessments of new members, and draw up special programmes for them with an air of expertise. Images of pert young bodies abound; no one can be left in any doubt that slim, toned and muscled is right, and overweight or middle-aged wobble is all wrong. Health clubs also have a habit of tying new members in to twelve-month contracts, which must be fully paid even by those who give up after three. This is quite business savvy, as they know perfectly well that the drop-out rate within a few months of joining is astronomical.

The real problem is how much physical activity we have lost from our everyday lives in the last 30 years or so, including our children's lives. We have become almost immobilised by modern transport, the modern workplace and our passive, gadget-driven leisure time. This is a striking change in the space of one generation. A trip to an expensive gym for a couple of hours a week is a drop in the ocean as compensation, though this does not stop members of the fitness industry promoting themselves as the rescuers of our health. Obesity experts argue that so little energy is burned during these occasional fitness sessions that they cannot meaningfully contribute to weight-loss. It is a tricky message. Some people will interpret it to mean that there is no point in taking exercise and nothing could be further from the truth. Our bodies thrive on physical activity; they get stronger, faster, more balanced, better slept and less depressed in response to it, and at any age. Yet, our modern, sedentary lifestyles encourage us to become alienated from our bodies, as if they were little more than transport for our heads.

It is important not to be coy about what most people really want. They want to be slim - with or without health as an added bonus. This is the victory of the advertising industry and the manufactured glamour of our celebrity culture. The cult of thinness is nothing new. It can be traced right back to ancient Greece with all its muscled Olympians and statuesque women in figure-hugging drapery. It can be seen again in the obsessive religious fasting of the Medieval period and the breath-restricting corsetry that bound women right into the 20th century. Victorian romanticism elevated pale, waif-like thinness, preferably to the point of fainting, to the height of gothic fashion; this applied to women as well as certain types of poetic men, such as Lord Byron. Indeed, waifs have had lasting appeal from the boyish flapper girls in the 1920s to the 'Twiggy' look of the 1960s. In modern times, 'heroin-chic' emaciation has been held up as a beauty ideal. Fortunately this seems to be passing out of fashion, though too many catwalk models are still painfully thin.

New heights of body fascism were scaled in the post-war years, and over the following, permissive decades. Never before had women had the freedom to expose so much flesh. Bikinis, swimsuits, miniskirts and shorts became ubiquitous on beaches and streets during the summer months. But freedom comes at a price, and today women are expected to reveal their bare legs, their arms, their midriffs, their cleavage, their backs and sometimes most of their buttocks. Furthermore, these should be slim, toned, tanned, shaved and cellulite free. Freedom from corsets was replaced by an obligation to achieve the same silhouette in the flesh. (In fact, we are returning to a form of corsetry with modern shaper garments and 'magic knickers' made of Spandex.) It is an impossible ideal for women to achieve. Yet for all the feminist rage against such tyranny, the belief that the fault lies with the woman who fails to achieve this ideal has taken root. Increasingly, it also applies to men.

For a long time, men were exempt from all this. They were free to strut around with beer bellies and 'man-boobs' without censure. This has changed in the last 20 years or so. Nowadays, men are also under pressure to have beautiful, youthful bodies with a six-pack, sculpted pectoral muscles and bulging biceps. Men's magazines emulate those for women by peddling images of physical perfection that are near impossible and exhausting to attain. And men face a doubly whammy; they are not allowed to be too thin either, with all its connotations of weakness.

For men and women, these manipulated, air-brushed images of physical perfection have become the unreachable benchmark of attractiveness. Even the models in the photographs don't actually look like that. Most of us know perfectly well that these images are lies, yet we still buy into their message, and feel judged when compared with them. If you are not convinced by how menacing these messages are, or the extent to which they have been internalised, let me spell them out below. As you read them, ask yourself how much you *know* them to be untrue on one hand, but at some level still *believe* them to be true on the other.

For women:

Slim is glamorous. Fat is frumpy and homely.

Slim is self controlled. Fat is out of control.

Slim is always attractive. Fat is never attractive.

Slim is success. Fat is failure.

Slim is superior. Fat is inferior.

For men:

Muscled is glamorous. Fat is homely. Skinny is feeble.

Muscled is disciplined. Fat is undisciplined. Skinny is weak.

Muscled is alpha-male. Fat or skinny is delta-male.

Muscled is driven and successful. Fat is lazy. Skinny is ineffectual.

Muscled is superior. Fat or skinny is inferior.

These messages are not just wrong, they are outrageous. Yet, if any of them caused you a spasm of anxiety then, somewhere along the line, they were successfully installed into your system of beliefs.

The advertising industry bombards us with images that associate female slimness and male muscle with success and attractiveness to force us to compare ourselves unfavourably with them. It then offers salvation in the form of the product it hopes you will buy: dieting books, slimming aids, low-calorie foodstuffs, gym membership, exercise equipment, etc. And we buy into it hook line and sinker. This is how advertising works, and it's all nonsense.

If the dieting and fitness industries were really selling workable solutions, why are we in the middle of an out-of-control obesity pandemic? At best, it could be argued their presence makes no difference. But the possibility that the dieting industry in particular is a contributing cause of obesity must be given serious consideration, especially with regard to rapid weight-loss diets. Furthermore, the images and messages of the advertising industry must be challenged. If this is a big ask for society, then at least it can be done at an individual level. If we reject slimness for slimness' sake as a beauty ideal, we become free to reinstate robust health as an achievable aim, and with it the real prospect of a better quality of life.

THE FOOD AND DRINKS INDUSTRY

Many experts blame the spread of fast food for the rise in obesity across the Western world and beyond. The post-war trends are difficult to ignore. During the Second World War, British food imports were severely reduced when German U-boats blockaded the Atlantic. Strict rationing was introduced putting the whole nation on a bland, stodgy diet of wholemeal bread, potatoes, oatmeal, and a lot of home-grown vegetables.

By today's standards, it was a low-fat diet with restrictions on dairy produce, meat, eggs, margarine and lard. The war effort galvanised the whole country; farming, munitions work and heavy industries were kept going, notably by women taking over the jobs of men fighting abroad. Add to this all the walking and cycling due to petrol rationing, and it is small wonder that the population became the fittest and healthiest it has ever been before or since. So what went wrong in the following decades?

Although sugared soda drinks, such as Coca-Cola, have been around since the late 1800s, most of the famous fast-food brands emerged in the USA in the 1950s. They have grown from strength to strength, and many of these brands are now a ubiquitous part of our global 'takeaway' culture. They include brands for hamburgers, deep-fried chicken, pizza, Mexican-style food, ice-cream, donuts, coffee bars, sandwich bars, cream cakes and pastries. Over the same period, big brand supermarkets have evolved to dominate our food supplies. They give us aisle after aisle of processed, convenience foods, along with soda drinks, crisps and snacks, cakes and biscuits, sugared cereals and, of course, cheap alcohol.

The march of this Western-style food across the world has also been linked to rising global trends in obesity. It is argued that this type of food has lured local populations away from their healthier, peasant dishes in South America, the Middle East, Russia, India, China, even Japan and parts of Africa. The truth is more complex. Over the centuries, rural diets in many developing countries were sparse and monotonous, often short of essential nutrients. The (mostly American) supermarket chains that have expanded into these territories offer a wide variety of affordable, safe food with production and storage standards that are quality controlled. It is little wonder they have been so successful. Brand-name fast-foods are also attractive to young people keen to associate themselves with Western trends, while they distance themselves from the old traditions.

Even such a brief overview highlights the tension between public health concerns and the might of the food and drink industries. These companies react aggressively towards any threat to their profits. In America, for example, many school districts have 'pouring rights' contracts with soft drink corporations. In exchange for large donations, that enable some struggling schools to buy essential equipment, they agree to sell only that company's products in school vending machines. Attempts to ban these products in schools by some public health boards were successfully challenged by the drinks companies in the courts.[10] Repeated attempts to stop fast-food companies in America from targeting children in their television advertising campaigns have also failed.

Schools in the UK have successfully banned soda-drink vending machines. Even the humble tuck shop is now a thing of the past. Despite these measures, and a UK ban on food adverts during children's television, we are all exposed to a constant stream of fast-food advertising. Pay attention to the internet, supermarkets, cinemas, high streets, shopping malls, train stations and airports, and you will see how extreme this has become.

The argument from the food and drinks industries is always the same; adults should be free to eat whatever they please, and parents are solely responsible for their children's diet. These companies say they are simply responding to demand, and are absolved of responsibility for the health risks associated with excessive consumption of their products. They see no reason why they should not be free to continue to market them aggressively. And as the vying and manoeuvring to protect profits continues, the world gets fatter and fatter.

So what is it about this type of food that links it so strongly to those who are overweight or obese? Well, for a start, it is abundant and highly palatable. Most of it is sold in excessively large portions, and has been packaged to make it easy to eat on the go, or while sitting in front of a TV or computer. Nearly all of it is extremely energy-dense (high-calorie). There are particular concerns about the high consumption of sugared soda drinks, sometimes called liquid candy, especially among children. These drinks seem to bypass our natural satiety mechanisms so can be consumed in volume without triggering the body's natural 'full' signals. There is also growing evidence that the 'diet' versions of these drinks may contribute to weight gain by triggering sugar cravings.[11] This has been disputed by research funded by the drinks companies.[12] This type of food appeals to almost everyone to a greater or lesser extent, but there may also be demographic factors involved.

Over the last forty to fifty years, more and more women have had to go out to work. This became a necessity as the economic landscape changed in the UK, and elsewhere, from the 1970s onwards. Today, only a minority of women have the option of remaining at home full time with their children. Inevitably, takeaway and convenience foods are going to be practical options for exhausted parents coping with the demands of raising children, running a home, and going out to work. Families sitting together for home-cooked meals are becoming a thing of the past.

UK census figures from 2011 show that single-person homes have risen to around 30% of households (18% in 1971), with a higher percentage in cities. More men than women under 65 live alone (58%), which possibly reflects the fact that children tend to live with their mothers after divorce.[13] It is a significant shift in the fabric of our society. It does not follow, of course, that someone will eat more convenience food or takeaways just because they live alone, but it is a demographic change that coincides with the rise in excess weight and obesity over the last forty years.

There is much disagreement between nutritional scientists about what constitutes an optimal diet, but there is strong consensus on some points. Firstly, we should all be eating far more vegetables than we currently do. We should also be increasing our intake of fruit but not at the expense of vegetables. Some nutritionists argue that we should be eating an essentially plant-based diet with only modest quantities of fish, poultry or meat. Secondly, it is widely agreed that we should greatly reduce the amount of processed food that we consume. But what exactly does 'processed' mean in this context, and is all processing bad?

Professor Carlos Monteiro, from The Centre of Nutrition at the University of Sao Paulo, Brazil, suggests three categories of processing to use as a general guide.[14] Clearly, fresh vegetables and fruit are unprocessed, but all otherwise perishable foods must be preserved in some way if it is not for immediate consumption.

Type 1 processing, according to Monteiro, does not substantially change the properties of the unprocessed food. The purpose is to extend shelf life with simple procedures such as parboiling, fermenting or sealing with aspic. This has been done for centuries and protected communities from starvation, especially during winter months. Meat, fish and game are dried, cured and smoked. Grain crops are threshed, milled, or malted. Milk is pasteurised to kill harmful bacteria, churned for butter, soured for yogurt or made into cheese. These processes produce fine foods. It could be argued that even the simplest cooking method from poaching an egg to adding yeast to flour counts as processing. Clearly, this type of minimal processing enhances food safety and variety, and need not concern us.

Type 2 processing creates culinary ingredients that would not normally be consumed on their own, such as oils, fats, refined grains and sugar. This category includes ingredients used by food and drinks manufacturers. Most of these products are acceptable but two are not: refined carbohydrates such as white flour or sugar; and hydrogenated fats, sometimes known as trans fats. Trans-fats are cheap and greatly extend the shelf-life of food. There is evidence, however, that they cause an elevation in levels of fat in the blood and so increase the risk of heart attack and stroke. They are found in many convenience foods and mass-produced bakery products.

Type 3 products are foods that are 'ready to eat' or 'ready to heat', at the point of purchase. Generally, these foods have been subjected to industrial levels of processing which have changed them significantly from their natural state. Monteiro introduces the term 'ultra-processed' to describe these products. For example, the protein remnants from animal carcasses that would otherwise be discarded can be mechanically recovered with high-pressure grinders and centrifuges. This produces a kind of slurry which, when mixed with various chemicals, can be reconstituted to look, smell and taste like slices of meat or 'nuggets' of poultry. Such products also contain many chemical preservatives and additives.

There are two groups of ultra-processed products. The first includes snacks such as crisps, sweets, chocolate bars, soft drinks and pre-packaged cakes and biscuits. The second group includes takeaway food such as burgers, fried chicken, pizza, donuts, etc, as well as 'ready-meal' products to be heated up at home. Monteiro is careful to point out that 'ultra-processed' products are not dangerous if consumed in moderation, the problem is one of proportion. He states:

"From the public health point of view, ultra-processed foods are problematic in two ways. First, their principal ingredients (oils, solid fats, sugars, salt, flours, starches) make them excessive in total fat, saturated or *trans*-fats, sugar and sodium, and short of nutrients and dietary fibre. Second, their high energy density, hyper-palatability, their marketing in large and super-sizes, and aggressive and sophisticated adverting, all undermine the normal processes of appetite control, which causes over-consumption and therefore obesity."[15]

Convenient, fast-food is typically around 65% higher in calories than its minimally processed equivalent, due to the added fat and sugar. Moreover, ultra-processed products are often consumed to the exclusion of fresh foods; lettuce with a burger is usually little more than trimming to give an illusion of wholesomeness. People who have become overweight or obese consuming these types of food are, therefore, often also suffering from a degree of malnutrition. This is of particular concern for growing children.

As a society, we have become alienated from the source of the food we consume. Although we love cookery programmes and recipe books, home cooking is rapidly disappearing as the norm of family life. Yet meals cooked from scratch are usually substantially lower in calories and higher in nutrients than ultra-processed foods. They are also far more economical. The ability to cook opens up a huge range of delicious meals that are otherwise sacrificed to dull 'dieting' food, or the monotony (let's be honest) of greasy, sugary or salty fast-foods.

What I hope to have demonstrated here is the extent to which we are in thrall to giant food and drinks manufacturers, and equally giant food retailers. We all need a degree of convenience in our busy lives, but I hope I have persuaded some readers to review their relationship with the modern food environment and, if necessary, take steps to reclaim this vital aspect of life.

DIRE HEALTH WARNINGS

The standard tactic of healthcare professionals, and government health departments, is to try to terrify people with threats of impending doom if they do not lose weight. Alarmist statistics also feature frequently in news reports and magazines. I am not convinced such scaremongering works. I face two problems drawing attention to this. Firstly, to make the point, I must highlight the health risks associated with obesity, and 1 may invoke the very fear to which I am objecting. Secondly, the health risks are real and not an illusion based on wrong beliefs. It is the scaremongering I take issue with, however, not the validity of the health evidence against obesity.

Most people who are significantly overweight are aware of the health risks. For example, it is well known that being overweight increases the likelihood of heart attack or stroke. One of the most common causes is high blood pressure; 66% of people with high blood pressure in the UK are overweight.[16] The risks are elevated further if excess fat is carried round the abdomen and/or in the presence of diabetes. Poor diet can also elevate the level of fat in the blood (especially damaging hydrogenated or trans-fats), which is associated with clogged-up arteries, and there is clear evidence that these damaging effects start at a young age.[17]

The incidence of type 2 diabetes is rising sharply, notably in young people, who will have to live with its difficult consequences for the rest of their lives. The risk of developing type 2 diabetes is about 20 times higher for people who are obese compared to those who are lean. Again, abdominal obesity is a particular risk. For reasons that are not well understood, diabetes is especially damaging to the circulatory system. Even when stabilised with diet and medication, people with diabetes are more prone to heart attacks and strokes. There is also a higher risk of kidney disease, impaired eyesight, poor skin healing, premature ageing and erectile dysfunction. There is a misconception that losing weight and good diet can cure type 2 diabetes. Sadly this is not correct, though these measures can contain the symptoms. Importantly, up to 80% of cases can be prevented or delayed with weight loss, exercise and good diet. (Visit www.diabetes.org.uk for more information.)

It is also known that people who are overweight or obese have a higher risk of developing cancer than those who are lean, though the reasons for this are complex and not fully understood. A recent UK study found that several cancers were linked to obesity, including cancers of the womb, gallbladder, kidney, bowel and liver. There is also an increased risk of post-menopausal breast cancer.[18]

People who are overweight or obese are also more prone to gallstones, liver failure, diverticular disease, and haemorrhoids as well as impaired mobility from worn-out arthritic joints and back pain. In addition to all this, there may be problems with excessive snoring or serious breathing problems during sleep. Women may have stress incontinence and/or vaginal prolapse. Worryingly, a recent study found that *uncorrected* obesity in younger life (from the 30s) also carries a much higher risk of dementia in later life.[19]

It is a frightening list. Healthcare professionals waving it at their overweight patients hope it will be a spur to action, but, if not handled carefully, it can make things worse. People who are overweight need to know about these risks, but I have often seen it make them feel even more miserable and scared than they were to start with. It intensifies their sense of powerlessness if they have failed to lose weight on many previous occasions. Moreover, it can leave them feeling bewildered, perhaps even a little stupid, when such obvious warnings are not enough to make them change. This is unfair. The journey to regaining health and a normal weight needs positive reinforcement, not a stoking of despair. The fear strategy has logic, but is nonetheless flawed.

We protect ourselves instinctively. We run from physical dangers, such as violence or fire, but also from psychological threats that are emotionally painful, frightening or humiliating. The list of health risks above poses such a psychological threat. Being confronted with it brings waves of anxiety that may seem overwhelming, so it is suppressed and depersonalised. Someone who is overweight may form a protective belief that these health risks only apply to other people who are overweight, and not to themselves. This is the protective mechanism of denial, and it is powerful. It subtly blocks the belief that personal action needs to be taken.

A health crisis, such as a heart attack, was one of the most common triggering events in those who finally succeeded in maintaining a normal weight. It was a sudden stripping away of their denial, clearly not a pleasant experience, which allowed them to see that these risks applied to them absolutely. The corrective action was immediate and permanent. This action, though, was not framed as a flight from fear but rather a steadfast reclaiming of health. This positive mindset is common in this group of people and I shall return to this theme frequently. It is worth noting, that there is strong evidence that long-term weight loss of just 5-10% reduces many of these health risks to a disproportionately greater extent, in particular high blood pressure.[20]

It seems that we live in a world that extols the delights of very fattening food, while blaming anyone for getting fat eating it, and then terrifying them about the health risks. But is it really possible to break out of this ghastly, imprisoning triangle? Is it possible to rise above the marketing, the junk food and the scaremongering, and carve your own path to normal weight and health? After years of dieting, of getting fatter and fatter, is this a realistic expectation? Frankly, yes it is, and in the next chapter I want to introduce some of the people who have done exactly that.

Achieving and Maintaining Long-Term Weight Loss

Most people tend to measure the success or failure of a diet by the lowest number they see on the weighing scales, before an all too predictable weight regain starts to take hold. Accolades are given to this diet or that diet in accordance with the total amount of weight lost, however briefly, but almost never to the length of time that weight loss was sustained. Surely this is a better gauge though? Is it not better to keep a few pounds off over a year than to lose a lot but regain more over a few months? It is certainly better for one's health. Yo-yo dieting (weight cycling) is almost as bad for health as being overweight in the first place.

People who manage to shed a lot of weight, and maintain that loss over time, are an elusive group who tend to fall off the research radar. This is a pity, for they are a vital source of information, especially against a background of escalating obesity. I felt their experiences could hold the key for many people who are overweight or obese and give them real hope that it was genuinely possible to do this. I thought their success would challenge some of the myths about being overweight or obese, which so many accept as incontrovertible truths. But first I had to find them.

I tracked down several studies about people who had sustained weight loss. I also took account of the personal weight-loss journeys given by authors in many diet books. Of particular interest was a book by Anne M Fletcher, *Thin for Life: 10 Keys to success from people who have lost weight and kept it off*, though this was published almost twenty years ago.[21] Fletcher interviewed 160 people who had achieved and maintained substantial weight loss and distilled this into common principles. This was useful but the numbers were relatively small.

It was my good fortune to find the National Weight Control Registry (NWCR), which was established by the University of Colorado in the USA in 1994 and is still going strong.[22] The NWCR represents the largest study being undertaken of long-term weight loss and currently tracks over 10,000 individuals who meet their criteria for joining. Members must be aged 18 or over, with a weight loss of 30 pounds or more that has been sustained for at least one year. In fact, most members have lost far more than this, and kept it off for much longer. The NWCR makes it clear, however, that they do not offer any weight-loss treatment programmes, nor do they give information or advice about weight loss.

SUCCESS RATES

Professors Rena Wing, James Hill and their colleagues, who set up the NWCR, define long-term weight loss as maintaining intentional weight loss of at least 10% for one year. In fact, members of the registry have lost an average of 66 lbs and kept this off for five and a half years. Their body mass index has fallen from an average of 36.7 kg/m^3 to 25.1 kg/m^3, just on 'healthy weight'.[23] Professor Wing states: "At one year follow-up, the majority of members had either maintained their weight loss (59%) or had lost additional weight (6%).".[24] Although some had regained weight (35%), this was not nearly as much as they had lost in the first place. According to the NWCR website, however, these averages conceal a lot of diversity. Weight loss ranges from 30 to 300 lbs, and timescales from one year to over six decades. These figures are eye-catching, but because NWCR members volunteered to register (rather than being randomly selected by researchers), they are not representative of the general overweight or obese population.

It is commonly believed that long-term weight loss is very difficult to achieve. Figures as low as 5% are often quoted in mainstream media but little evidence supports this. Someone wanting to lose weight may feel the odds are stacked against them from the start. I was keen to track down more accurate figures, but studies on this subject are sparse.

Wing and Hill believe the weight-loss success rate is actually about 20%, using a definition of 10% weight loss held down for at least a year (not lost over one year).[25] Other studies provide an even better picture. One study tracked the weight loss of 621 people. At 3-year follow-up 53% had maintained a 5% weight loss; a further 35% sustained a loss of 10% or more.[26] Another study, with 154 participants, found that 40% were maintaining a weight loss of 5% at five years; and 25% were maintaining a 10% loss seven years later.[27] These may seem like modest decreases in weight but it should be remembered that a sustained weight loss of just 5-10% is associated with significant health benefits.

THE TRIGGERING EVENT

Most of the studies I reviewed, and most dieting books, focus exclusively on the behaviours that resulted in long-term weight loss, rather than motivation. They discuss what foods were eaten or avoided and how much exercise was taken. These behaviours are a response to motivation, however, and, if this is not taken into account, a vital piece of the overall picture is missing.

As I read through the testimonials and studies, it became clear that the common denominator of these success stories was a determined mindset that was quite different from anything experienced before. Nearly all of these people spoke of some event that suddenly altered their perspective on the importance of regaining their health. It is in such moments that deeply held beliefs about weight or health evaporate. New possibilities open up that seemed closed off before.

Many of these triggering events were health scares, but most were not. In fact, a lot of them would seem rather inconsequential to someone else. Nevertheless, they struck such a deep chord within the individual concerned that they changed their behaviours almost immediately. I will discuss this aspect of suddenly altered beliefs tripping into life-changing behaviours in more detail in the next chapter.

Although my emphasis is on the power of beliefs, I am aware that readers hoping to lose weight will also be interested in the techniques and strategies used by those who succeeded in maintaining significant weight loss, so I have included them below.

WEIGHT-LOSS AND MAINTENANCE STRATEGIES

For the sake of ease, I shall now refer to those who have sustained a lower weight as 'maintainers'. Sifting through the studies and books, it was possible to identify key principles that most maintainers stuck to in order to reach their health and weight goals. They are entirely predictable. They will not surprise veteran dieters, who may even be disappointed if they have tried these approaches in the past to no avail. I believe this confirms that it is the right mindset that makes the real difference in the long-term.

The maintainers made permanent changes to their entire lifestyle, not just their diet. There was a strong commitment to making good decisions about food and exercise for life, and complete acceptance of this from the outset, even when faced with an occasional set back.[28] This was in contrast to many failed attempts to lose weight in the past. This aspect of long-term weight loss is conspicuously absent from most diet books or regimes, many of which promise a one-off cure for fatness. They imply that weight loss is a temporary exercise that can be separated from the rest of one's life. With such a short-term view, however, the pre-diet lifestyle will likely be resumed and weight regained. Those who weight-cycle (yo-yo) fall into this trap again and again.

This may bother some readers. It suggests that long-term weight loss means a life deprived of favourite foods, and an ongoing struggle with fragile willpower. It is not so. Maintainers consistently reported a sense of liberation, and a marked improvement in the quality of their lives. Their experiences were expressed strongly in terms of what they had gained, not what they had lost; they gained freedom, a healthy weight and nourishing food. I found no reports where maintainers expressed unhappiness because they missed junk food. These 'gain' attitudes prevailed over any sense of deprivation or sacrifice. There is also evidence that weight maintenance gets easier over time. The likelihood of long-term success starts to increase after a year, and continues to improve.[29]

FOOD STRATEGIES

Nearly all maintainers designed their own weigh-loss plan. Experienced dieters tend to know what does or does not work for them, so can tailor a plan to their specific needs, lifestyle and budget.[30] According to the NWCR, 45% of maintainers lost weight on their own; the other 55% had some sort of support, such as joining a slimming club or getting one-on-one help from a psychotherapist or dietician.[31] Due to urgent health needs, a few dropped their weight quite quickly but the majority lost weight gradually, in a few cases over as many as 14 years. This meant creating a sustainable plan that could be integrated into their lives for good.

89% of maintainers used a combination of food management as well as physical activity. Only 10% used diet alone and just 1% used only physical activity.[32] In the last 10 years carbohydrate-restricted diets have become more popular, reflecting the shift in evidence discussed in the previous chapter. More recently, a trend for intermittent fasting has emerged. This involves eating very little (500-600 calories) every other day or on alternate days, or eating only within the same 8-hour period each day. This is just another way to cut calories per week but supporters argue in favour of its sustainability. None of the maintainers I studied had used intermittent fasting, but their weight loss predates the recent popularity of this regime.

Nearly all the maintainers ate regular meals, especially breakfast (78%). A consistent weekly pattern of eating was followed, and meals and shopping were carefully planned to maintain vigilance over the calorie content of each meal.[33] This vigilance was sustained during holidays and social occasions, pointing to the ongoing commitment to health regardless of circumstances. Many people regard these events as excuses to overeat. We have been conditioned to associate socialising and celebration with overeating, though it is obviously possible to enjoy these activities without consuming excessive amounts of food or drink. I will return to this theme in the next chapter.

Few maintainers excluded entire food groups, but they all greatly reduced their intake of energy-dense foods (sugary, fatty foods). They ate predominantly home-cooked food, and rarely ate convenience, takeaway or junk food. The switch to home-cooked meals is important. As a rule, meals cooked from scratch have considerably fewer calories than their ready-meal or fast-food equivalents. You also know exactly what is in a homemade meal, and what is not in it; there is no excess salt, no hidden sugar, no E-number flavourings or preservatives. If made with fresh produce, home-cooked meals are more nourishing and higher in fibre than ultra-processed ready-meals. With smart shopping, they are a lot cheaper too. And they taste so much better! We are gradually losing cookery skills as a society, but the ability to cook is an essential life skill. It is no accident that so many lean people are good home cooks; the maintainers seemed to have discovered this too.

Energy levels are boosted quite quickly when a poor diet of ultra-processed food is replaced by nourishing food. Physical activity becomes easier. A lot of people also find that their mood is lifted and stabilised. I am always puzzled when someone is surprised to discover that good food has this effect. It is an obvious win-win situation. Unsurprisingly, the maintainers reported a greater pleasure in food for its own sake, and the physical wellbeing that came with it, independently of feelings about weight.[34]

Maintainers paid attention to portion control. As a society we have become accustomed to excessive portions, notably from fast-food outlets and cinemas. Buffet-style restaurants that offer unlimited food for a fixed price have also become popular, and encourage customers pile their plates high. Even the muffins in high-street coffee shops are bigger than tennis balls. It is easy to see why so many people are not sure what an appropriate portion of food actually looks like anymore. And 'portions' can be subtly increased by grazing during cooking or eating the leftovers on a child's plate. Most maintainers had to weigh food until their eyes adjusted to correct portions.

Another common strategy used by the maintainers was to avoid situations where temptation would be strong. Snacks, sweets and soda drinks were kept out of the house, and family members were asked to understand why it had to be that way. One study found that those able to refuse 'food offerings' had a better chance of sustaining weight loss. This was associated with higher self-esteem and assertiveness; they were able to say no to someone pushing food at them.[35] This is an important topic. It ties into the associations we make between food and concepts of giving and receiving as well as anxiety about causing offence to others. I will return to this topic in the next chapter.

It is worth mentioning that most naturally lean people balance their food intake over a few days, or even over an entire week. A subtle mental record is kept of food consumed, or due to be consumed, so that compensations can be factored in. Lunch may be skipped if a restaurant meal is planned in the evening; a side-serving of potatoes may be dropped at supper to balance out that morning's Danish pastry, and so on. This is done quite automatically without the need to count calories. People who have been a normal, healthy weight throughout life know how much these small adjustments matter. A lot of maintainers seem to gradually develop the confidence to do this once their new pattern of eating has become established, though it can take a bit of practice.

PHYSICAL ACTIVITY

Nearly all maintainers engaged in physical activity to keep their weight down. Regular brisk walking was the most popular activity with NWCR members (76%), followed by cycling (20%), weight resistance training (20%) and aerobic classes (18%). Women preferred walking and aerobics; men preferred competitive sports and weight lifting.[36]

One study divided 45 previously obese participants into three activity groups to assess the impact of exercise on weight-loss maintenance over two years. The groups were:

- low-level activity (under 850 kcals per week), walking less than half an hour a day

- moderate activity (850-1575 kcals per week), walking 30-45 minutes per day

- high-level activity (over 1575 kcals per week), walking over 45 minutes per day

Most walked briskly as their preferred activity. Unsurprisingly, the high-level activity group maintained significantly greater weight loss than the other groups. They also had a greater reduction in blood cholesterol levels, which lowers the risk of heart attack and stroke.[37]

Brisk walking is excellent for general health. It provides aerobic exercise, tones muscles and increases bone density all in one go. It is eminently suited to those wanting to lose weight. Walking doesn't need expensive gym membership, cumbersome equipment or flesh-revealing clothes. It also protects the self-conscious from the flushing, sweating and wobbling of jogging in public. Brisk walking burns roughly the same number of calories as jogging, it just takes longer to cover the same distance. All you have to do is step out of your front door and start. Exercise like this is an underrated antidepressant and mood-enhancer, whether you need to lose weight or not. This is partly biochemical but it is also great stress-breaker in its own right. If life is hectic, it's great to get out for some fresh air.

Obesity experts have recently cast doubt on exercise as a weight-reducing strategy because the calories burned in a single gym session are so modest. I want to clarify this. It is true to say that exercise alone, without adjustment to food intake, results in limited weight-loss; it is the combination which works so well. The relevance of exercise to weight loss is not about a calculation of calories burned versus calories eaten on a day-to-day basis. It is about muscle. Our bodies love muscle and it is vital to our health. Muscle burns more energy than other body tissues, so increasing its mass increases the metabolic rate. This makes a real difference over time. This is part of the long-game of weight loss, and it is more important than calorie number-crunching on the day. This is why maintainers who do specific weight-resistance training have an advantage.

People tend to think that weight-resistance training means pumping iron but many activities count, such as yoga and Pilates. Although muscle degenerates with age if not used to capacity, this can be reversed with sufficient weight-resistance exercise. Skeletal muscle is a malleable tissue that can be built up with specific activities. Remarkably, muscle reverts to a more youthful state if weight-resistance exercise is maintained.

One study found that mobility, balance and independence improved in a group of elderly nursing-home residents after exercising with free weights for six months. They also had fewer falls.[38] Another study demonstrated that older people over the age of 60 can regenerate and build muscle to the same bulk and strength of people in their 20s, though they have to work harder to maintain this.[39]

Finally, there is *non-exercise activity thermogenesis*, thankfully known as NEAT for short. This jargon phrase refers to all the energy we burn that is not eating, sleeping or formal exercise. It includes gardening, cooking, taking a shower, even fidgeting. Physically demanding jobs, such as those involving manual labour, have high NEAT, whereas someone sitting at a computer all day will have low NEAT. This general day-to-day activity has a big impact on body weight, and it is quite easy to increase. Many people are familiar with this advice, for example: climb stairs instead of taking the lift; get off a bus a few stops early and walk; cycle or walk short journeys instead of taking the car. All this movement adds up. People who are lean tend to have high NEAT. There are many ways to make daily life more active, and some of these simple changes are a good starting point for people who have not done formal exercise for some time.

I hope that I have made a good case for the importance of physical activity. As strength and energy increase, so too will the desire to remain active, as though the extra energy itself generates a restless impulse to move. Interestingly, Anne Fletcher noted that many of her interviewees were instinctively drawn to healthy foods when they increased their activity levels, as if by some alchemy the two simply went together.

THE RISK OF REGAIN

People who have been on many diets over the years know how easy it is to regain the weight that was lost. It is immensely frustrating. The highest risk of weight regain is within the first year after losing weight but then the risk recedes. Those reaching the 2-year milestone have a much greater chance of maintaining long-term weight loss and a near guarantee of it at five years.[40]

It is not surprising that the core reason for weight regain is giving up the behaviours that brought about the weight loss in the first place. When dietary vigilance falls, the consumption of fat, sugar and fast food rises. Physical activity drops and more time is spent watching television. (62% of NWCR members watch less than ten hours of television per week.) Those who regained weight were more likely to skip breakfast, snack on fattening foods and overeat at mealtimes. They were more likely to overeat when friends were overeating, and more likely to stock fattening snacks and drinks at home. They also found it difficult to refuse food that was offered to them by others.[41]

Maintainers weighed themselves frequently; there was a clear connection between this habit and keeping weight down. A study from the NWCR shows that more than 75% of members weighed themselves at least once a week.[42] Researchers in another study found that frequent self-weighing helped maintainers to catch small weight gains and nip them in the bud. Weight regain was much lower at one-year follow-up in participants who monitored their weight closely. Those who stopped frequent weighing were more likely to gradually increase their calorie and fat intake and disregard the impact of bouts of overeating.[43]

Maintainers set achievable targets. There is evidence that those who regain weight often set themselves weight targets that are too low. Unrealistic expectations are common. One study suggests that failure to reach their perfect weight may actually encourage someone to completely abandon the effort to maintain any weight loss. It is an all-or-nothing approach, but very few people reach their perfect lower weight.[44]

Nearly all maintainers regained a few pounds from their lowest weight but managed to hold things steady at that point. Few, however, recovered from regains of over 4 to 5 lbs; evidence suggests this is likely to trigger a much bigger regain. Any substantial break in their diet led to sustained overeating or binge eating, and those who regained all the weight they lost struggled to re-lose it the following year.[45]

In contrast, all successful long-term maintainers had pre-planned strategies for handling small weight gains that were implemented quickly. Firstly, they did not panic or fall into despair. They quickly forgave themselves for the occasional lapse and corrected this by cutting back over the next few days. Importantly, they didn't just give up. This distinguishes maintainers from those who are more rigid and unforgiving. Inflexibility is difficult to sustain and, ironically, seems to make weight regain more likely.[46]

Maintainers found non-food ways of dealing with stress and had more self-compassion. This helped prevent small regains of weight from turning into larger relapses. It should be remembered that the great majority of maintainers lost weight gradually, making it much easier to correct the regain of a few pounds.

It is known that depression interferes with the motivation needed to sustain any major lifestyle change, such as achieving and maintaining weight loss.[47] This strengthens the case for physical activity which is a mood-enhancer, but anyone suffering from depression that is disrupting daily life must see a doctor. Depression is a treatable illness. Once this is under control, it will be much easier to take steps to regain physical health too.

MYTH BUSTING

When Anne Fletcher interviewed 160 maintainers, she discovered they contradicted some commonly held beliefs about losing weight. These beliefs are generally held to be truths but are in fact myths.

If you have been overweight since childhood, it is impossible to lose weight and keep it off.

45% of Fletcher's interviewees had been overweight children and a further 25% had gained weight as teenagers.

They had all managed to lose weight in adulthood and had maintained this for several years.

If you have dieted and failed many times, there is little hope of ever succeeding in losing weight for good.

Nearly 60% of these maintainers had lost and regained weight on more than five previous occasions before finally succeeding. A further 20% had tried to lose weight three or four times. When it came to the final attempt, they had gained enough experience to know what did and did not work for them. Nearly all of them drew up their own individual weigh-loss plans on the strength of this.

If you succeed in losing weight and keeping it off, you will have to eat like a bird for the rest of your life.

Fletcher's maintainers ate regular meals every day and eventually gained enough flexibility to be able to enjoy the odd snack. 'Everything is moderation' is a core rule they came to understand. They all switched to a wholesome, nutritious diet and this opened up a whole new way of thinking about food. It became one of life's real pleasures instead of a problem. People who constantly weight-cycle may only know strict dieting or compulsive overeating – famine or feast - but a maintenance diet is around 2000 kcals per day and, compared to strict dieting, this is quite a generous amount of food.

In order to maintain weight loss, you have to become an exercise fanatic.

It was rare for the maintainers to engage in extreme levels of exercise. Nevertheless, 90% of NWCR members exercise for around 1 hour each day, most of which is walking. Around 70% of Fletcher's interviewees exercised three or more times a week, again with walking being the most popular activity. So, physical activity is extremely important but excessive amounts are quite unnecessary.

It is really difficult to lose weight past the age of 40.

At the NWCR, the average women is 45 and the average man is 49 (as opposed to the average overall age). Many of Fletcher's interviewees had also been over 40 when they started to lose weight for the final time, some were even in their 60s. There is no evidence that aging, of itself, causes a drop in metabolic rate, except in much later life. In particular, there is no evidence that menopause is a direct cause of weight gain. It is true that most people gain weight as they age but the strongest contributing factor is an increasingly sedentary lifestyle. Staying active keeps this at bay.

I was intrigued by the power of these myths. They confirm that we accept certain beliefs as truths when they are not. The maintainers dismissed them and successfully lost weight. The beliefs we hold set the direction of our lives to an extent that few people realise. They cascade into thoughts, feelings and behaviours, however unconsciously. Incorrect beliefs will adversely influence the course of our lives.

The great majority of maintainers identified a triggering event that dispelled or altered previously held beliefs. They were life-changing. They brought an entirely fresh perspective to the matter of achieving a normal weight and reclaiming health. It is to this that I now turn my attention.

Core Beliefs and Triggering Events

WHAT IS A TRIGGERING EVENT?

A triggering event is a pivotal moment of insight that alters or dispels a previously held belief and replaces it with a new perception about some or all aspects of life. Typically these moments seem sudden. They may be obviously dramatic, such as a brush with death, but are just as likely to arise through some commonplace experience, such as a passing conversation, reading a newspaper article, or seeing an image of something. Such moments resonate deeply with the individual concerned, and give rise to a new revelation or understanding about something.

Some people describe these events as epiphanies, as they cause such ruptures in their previously held view of the world. I use the word 'epiphany' with some caution because of its religious connotations. The magnitude of these experiences, however, can warrant the use of such a strong word. It is reasonable to apply it to sudden shifts of thinking on any aspect of life, such as health or politics, rather than using it solely for experiences that are spiritual or mystical.

People who have had such epiphanies often say there is no going back. It seemed to open a one-way door that they were compelled to go through, before it closed behind them. An insight, once seen, cannot be unseen. Fresh beliefs changed their thinking, feelings and behaviours almost immediately, and it altered the course of their lives.

There is an important distinction between this kind of belief-altering experience and temporary moments of resolve that are induced by anxiety. Many people get upset when they gain a lot of weight; they react by starting another weight-loss project with gusto and high hopes. As this becomes difficult to sustain, the diet and exercise plans start to peter out, weight starts to creep back on, and they go back to square one. The problem is that they are trying to implement big lifestyle changes while still adhering to the beliefs that led them to be overweight in the first place. In contrast, people who had a complete change of insight about their health, felt their new mindset carried them along their journey towards a normal weight.

Almost everyone has experienced moments of profound change at some point; they can affect all areas of life, not just health. It may be worth recalling their impact, especially if the distinction I make above is difficult to grasp. The following examples may help. (The characters I describe throughout this book are composites of people I have known or supported over the years.)

About ten years ago, Dianne, a young maths teacher, accepted a position at a large inner-city high school, which had known discipline problems. She was determined to keep her classes in order, so she took a tough stance with pupils who stepped out of line. Even though she worked hard to sustain this, she was still shocked by the level of anger and hostility she faced from some of the teenagers, especially the boys. They gave back-chat, disrupted the class and were pointedly uninterested in maths. Dianne pushed her hard-line approach but as the months went by things just got worse. Then one day, after a particularly difficult class, she lost her temper with one of the boys. She told him it was pointless trying to teach him anything and that she doubted he would ever amount to much. To her surprise, he burst into tears. He asked her why she was always such a bully. He wanted to know why she hated boys so much and why she never stopped shouting at them. As Dianne took in what he had said, she suddenly realised it was her own behaviour that was causing the disruption in her classes. The pupils were not being hostile towards her; they were defending themselves against her. She was harder on the boys because she was more afraid of them. Dianne felt ashamed of how mean she had been to them. No wonder they didn't want to learn anything from her. The teenage boy made Dianne see herself as others saw her, and she was appalled.

This incident changed Dianne's career, not just her classes. From that day on, she stopped being afraid of her pupils, and found the confidence to give them the respect and encouragement they deserved. Dianne is still a dedicated teacher working with under-privileged children.

Joe is in his 40s and works in London. He is a journalist. A late-starter, Joe took many menial, low-paid jobs right into his 30s before getting his career off the ground. For most of his life, Joe believed that attending college and building a career were beyond him. He had not done well at school and had received little encouragement at home. The direction of his life started to change, however, after a conversation with one of the managers at the factory where he worked. The manager noticed that Joe was becoming depressed and wanted to help. He told Joe that he often wondered why such a clever guy had so little ambition. Joe dismissed this comment but the manager persisted. Others had also noticed this, he said, and thought he could do anything he wanted. For the first time, Joe questioned his assumption that his abilities were limited. He realised he had no idea what he was really capable of because he had never applied himself to anything, and he became curious about his own potential.

Joe's depression lifted and he was given promotion at the factory. A year later he started a college degree which eventually led to his successful career as a journalist.

His life changed direction after one conversation because it forced him to challenge the beliefs he had about his abilities, and there was no going back.

These were triggering events for Dianne and Joe, even though the incidents themselves may seem insignificant to others. They caused shifts in thinking and behaviour that altered the course of their lives forever. Neither could have returned to their old ways of thinking even if they had wanted to. A new approach to life became inevitable and good outcomes followed.

Many of us can identify at least one similar moment from our own lives. If this applies to you, ask yourself if you could go back to the old way of thinking and behaving. If not, this was a triggering event in your life. It is quite different from speculatively trying a new behaviour, such as a new diet, and hoping it will work. It is also different from rationally drawing a conclusion about something, for, odd as it seems, it is possible to know something without quite believing it. For example, most smokers know that cigarettes are bad for health, yet they continue to smoke because they do not believe this applies to them.

Although most triggering events seem to have a sudden impact, they can also be more slow-burning yet just as effective. In their book, *Quantum Change: when epiphanies and sudden insights transform ordinary lives*, William Millar and Janet C'de Baca identify individuals who experienced fundamental, life-altering shifts in beliefs as a series of 'aha' realizations. These built up into a crescendo of insight about a particular area of their lives. Millar and C'de Baca concluded that the speed of such insights are not as important as their depth and impact.[48]

I agree up to a point. With the exception of an unexpected health crisis, I believe that most triggering events are preceded by a period where obstructing beliefs are being questioned by the mind, even if this is being done subconsciously. There is some awareness that the overall picture of life is not quite right. Dianne knew that she had not found the solution to the disruption in her classes, and sought to address this, albeit incorrectly, by applying greater discipline. Joe was succumbing to depression. There was a build up of 'not-rightness' that predisposed them to a triggering event.

THE TRIGGERING EVENTS OF WEIGHT-LOSS MAINTAINERS

I was keen to find out if there was a pattern to the triggering events experienced by people who had lost substantial amounts of weight and maintained this over time. Professor Rena Wing, Dr Amy Goran and Dr Suzanne Phelan from the National Weight Control Registry (NWCR) carried out a study of 917 registry members, all of whom had sustained at least 30 lbs of weight loss for around seven years. They found that 83% had experienced a definable triggering event that enabled them to do this, even though nearly all of them had tried and failed so many times before.[49, 50]

The largest single group were those who had experienced medical triggers (23%), such as having a heart attack or stroke. Medical triggers also included being told bluntly by a doctor that there was an imminent risk to health if weight was not reduced immediately. Some saw a close friend or family member become very ill or die due to an obesity-related cause. Other medical triggers include: needing medication for high blood pressure before the age of 40; or a perilous condition known as 'metabolic syndrome' that includes high blood sugar, high blood cholesterol and high blood pressure due to excess weight, especially around the abdomen – a health cliff edge. In her book *Thin for Life: 10 keys to success from people who have lost weight and kept it off*, Anne Fletcher gives an account of a man who had not been especially bothered by his 475 lb frame until he fell into water and almost drowned because he could not save himself. He went on to lose 250 lbs and kept it off.

These people had their denial about the risks of being overweight or obese suddenly torn away. They became very scared; not a pleasant experience but certainly a powerful one. They finally understood that they might actually die from the consequences of being so overweight but also, vitally, that it was not too late to do something about it.

The NWCR researchers found that more men than women reported medical triggers, and that they tended to be older (around 50 years of age) than those with non-medical triggers. It is known that the risks of these weight-related health problems rise with age. This group of maintainers had also lost on average 10 lbs more than those with non-medical triggers (80 lbs compared to 70 lbs), although most had been heavier to start with.[51] In a later study, the same researchers found that two years after joining the registry, members who had had a medical triggering event were more likely to have succeeded in keeping their weight right down than those with non-medical triggers. This testifies to the potency of these particular wake-up calls.[52]

Non-medical triggering events were also powerful and were, collectively, the largest category. For example, 21.3% finally lost weight for good after reaching an all time high weight. One member said: "I stepped on the scales and saw that I had reached 200 lbs for the first time in my life." Others saw a photo of themselves, or looked at themselves in a mirror, and were finally forced to see how out of hand things had become (12.7%). One woman suffered the indignity of her children playing the video of her 40th birthday party over and over again, and had to look at her obese self wearing a T-shirt saying "This is what 40 looks like!". She became determined it was not going to be what 45 looked like. Lifestyle factors, such as approaching a significant birthday, or applying for a new job were the triggers for 9%. Others reacted to social factors, such as being teased by a colleague or hearing others making remarks about their weight (7%).[53]

Anne Fletcher identified similar triggering events as the spurs to long-term weight loss, during her interviews of 160 successful maintainers. One man said: "I couldn't take it anymore. I was sick and tired of being self-destructive, of being overweight and feeling limited by my weight." He went on to lose 45 lbs, and kept it off for 20 years. Another said: "I was tired of having food run my life. Enough was enough." She lost 50 lbs and maintained this for six years. Fletcher also identified some maintainers who, having lost a significant amount of weight, enjoyed their new slim frame so much they became absolutely determined to keep it – a sort of delayed triggering event. Finally, there were maintainers who had ulterior motives for losing weight, like wanting to find a new partner.[54]

WHAT TRIGGERS A TRIGGERING EVENT?

William Miller and Janet C'de Baca noticed that sudden shifts in beliefs - 'quantum change' as they call it - came to those who were in some way looking out for this, even if they were not fully aware of it at the time. These individuals had not been brooding miserably about a problem in a swell of self-pity, rather they had been contemplating the root cause of a problem and had been scanning for solutions, often for a considerable period of time. This seemed to predispose them to a triggering event. It is as though there is a critical mass of questioning and searching that creates the seedbed for a triggering event in the mind. This openness makes it possible for the mind to respond to solutions presented to it from the social environment, or from personal wisdom.

Awareness of a life picture that seems wrong in some way is an important part of the process, even though it is uncomfortable when there is no obvious solution. Many people push such discomfort away, afraid they will slide into despair or excessive anxiety. Some use distracting activities to paper over the sense of powerlessness they feel when faced with what seems like an unsolvable problem. There is a hope that constant busyness will somehow bury the issue without them having to actually address it. It rarely works. It just continues to grind away relentlessly in the background, wearing them down.

Key precursors for a triggering event, then, are acceptance that some aspect of life is out of kilter, and a lasting desire for change. Importantly, the desire for change must prevail even when it is not known how this change will come about. The problem is held in the mind constructively without self-pity or avoidance. This ongoing contemplation is often just barely within conscious thought. It creates a receptive state of mind that constantly scans for answers: a heightened sensitivity to the world that seems to invite solutions. In this state, the mind will latch on to things of particular relevance that it might otherwise have dismissed, until there is a final shift in perspective. There is an immediacy to these moments. They bring sudden insights that appear to be out of the blue – a triggering event.

These triggering events, or epiphanies, are highly personal. What works for one person may have no effect on others. It shows how different we all are. Our beliefs about life, and about ourselves, are formed during childhood and from our unique experiences in life. While it is possible to identify common themes, no two people will hold the same beliefs. At the very least, we all use different words to describe our beliefs. Language is the powerful medium through which our beliefs are created, sustained and expressed.

Beliefs that have been held for a long time can be difficult to identify. They have often been accepted so completely they become confused with truth. Because of this, even strong beliefs are often hidden within plain sight. If someone is aware that something is not right about the of direction their life, but is at a loss to understand why, there are likely to be obstructing beliefs at play. A triggering event will expose a belief and bring it into full view. Sometimes just the knowledge of it is the cure. If not, at least such exposure allows a belief to be scrutinised and questioned.

In the examples above, both Dianne and Joe knew something was not right. Dianne was vexed at her inability to control her disruptive pupils, and had spent a lot of time trying to figure out the reasons for their hostility. It was only when one of them pointed out that she had become a bully that the whole picture came into sharp focus. Dianne had forgotten to look at herself because she had not thought there was anything wrong with her behaviour. If her mind had not been scanning for answers, she would probably have dismissed the boy's remarks as impertinence and carried on as before.

Joe had known for some time that he was drifting through life working in low-paid jobs. This distinguished him from most of his co-workers who all had different reasons for doing the same work: they were raising young families; paying their way through college; doing uncomplicated work before retiring; or gaining work experience after leaving school. He wanted to change his situation but couldn't see any way of doing so. It was not until his manager had that pivotal conversation with him that he questioned his assumptions about his own abilities.

Nearly all of the weight-loss maintainers had a history of failure that left them asking if there was a better way of doing things. Questioning the standard solution to being overweight seemed to set the scene for their triggering events. In her book, *Epiphany: True Stories of Sudden Insight to Inspire, Encourage, and Transform*, Elise Ballard, interviewed a woman, who had tried and failed to lose weight from her 300 lb frame many times. She finally realised it was her mind that needed to change, and she resolved to stop dieting until she found a new way of looking at the problem. In fact she prayed for help, which is a form of scanning, for several weeks. Her triggering event was watching a short television interview of a woman who started to lose weight by walking for one hour a day. She knew at once that this was something she could do too, so she walked out of her front door, kept going for thirty minutes, turned round and came back again. She did this every day. Her weight started to fall and she lost 140 lbs in 18 months, which she had maintained for three years.[55]

Ballard interviewed 58 people, from all walks of life. They described their epiphanies and the impact they had on their lives. In spite of their very different backgrounds, Ballard noticed common threads that ran through all of their stories, as follows:

1. LISTENING. Whether they were calmly contemplating the sky, meditating or praying,

clinging to hope in a crisis, desperate to heal, or searching for an answer, people were listening and paying attention to signs and what was going on around them.

2. BELIEF. When people had an epiphany, they never doubted for one instant the significance of what had happened. [It] was real for them.

3. ACTION. Every single person whose epiphany positively changed his or her beliefs took action. All of them took steps toward whatever the epiphany compelled them to do.

4. SERENDIPITY. After people began to take action on their epiphanies, circumstances seemed to fall into place so that they could take the next step.. as if the world conspired to support [their] actions and confirm [they were] on the right track.

Many (not all) of Ballard's interviewees felt their experience had a strong spiritual element, as if there were some benevolent force operating on their behalf. Miller and C'de Baca also made a distinction between 'quantum change' that seemed to have a mystical element and those that were simply insightful. Predictably, those who had a religious faith were more likely to have spiritual experiences than others.[56]

One of the best known calls to faith is from Alcoholics Anonymous (AA), though the organisation scrupulously avoids endorsing any particular religion. Recovering alcoholics talk about 'hitting bottom', and the AA recognises this as an essential step to sobriety – the AA equivalent of a triggering event. It is seen as the critical low point from which two paths diverge: one swirling down into chaos and death; the other offering life, hope and stability. In contrast to the usual encouragement to 'pull yourself together', the AA asks for complete surrender to a higher power in the quest for sobriety. The alcoholic must recognise his or her powerlessness to achieve this alone.[57] The success of AA since its inception 80 years ago is well documented.

It is probable that people with a strong spiritual faith will find this a particular source of support as they address their difficulties with being overweight or obese. It is by no means a necessary condition of experiencing a triggering event or epiphany, however, nor is any kind of spiritual faith an inevitable consequence of it.

THE IMPACT OF A TRIGGERING EVENT

Ballard noted that people who have had an epiphany, whether insightful or spiritual, have strong convictions about the validity of their new view of the world. They believed in it, and felt immediately compelled to act in accordance with it. I noticed a similar quality in the accounts of the weight-loss maintainers that I came across during my own research. There was a new steel in the final attempt to lose weight that had been absent from previous attempts. Many maintainers said they "just knew" that this time they would pull it off for good. They made a fundamental decision to change the way they lived their lives from then on.

Maintainers spoke of making these big changes in their lives for themselves, sometimes explicitly saying that it no longer mattered what anyone else thought. One of Anne Fletcher's interviewees described it as similar in magnitude to a religious conversion.[58] With such strong convictions, it is hardly surprising that success rates within this group were so high and long lasting.

Ballard also noted that many of her interviewees experienced what seemed like a strange serendipity in the weeks and months after their epiphanies. They had additional mini-revelations or unexpected coincidences which seemed to offer further support for their journey. When Millar and C'de Baca asked their respondents when they thought their 'quantum change' triggering event had ended, nearly all stated that it hadn't. In some way, they each felt it had continued ever since.

I can see why some people wonder if such serendipity has a mystical cause, and perhaps it does. My own view is that the openness of mind that created the readiness for a triggering event in the first place continues to scan for relevant information. We are exposed to a huge amount of information every day from all sorts of directions. If you tried to take it all in you would go a little mad, so your brain selects only the information it needs or wants and filters out the rest. If a triggering event has created a heightened awareness about something specific, your brain will pluck useful morsels of information from your surroundings and present them to you, instead of blotting them out. It does not matter much if you believe this is some kind of spiritual intervention or simply a feature of your remarkable brain; either way, it is delightful and worth cultivating.

THE CENTRAL ROLE OF BELIEFS

Ask someone about their beliefs and it will be assumed you are asking about religious beliefs. We hold strong beliefs about all areas of our lives, however, and they determine how we view and engage with the world. Great or small, our beliefs affect how we think and act every day. Obstructive beliefs can only be changed if they are identified, tested and reconstructed. This is rarely a matter of simply deciding to believe something different – beliefs are more tenacious than that – but it is a matter of preparing your mind for your own triggering event. First, though, you need to know what those beliefs are.

Religion aside, the main beliefs you hold should be fairly easy to identify. When people talk about their moral values, they really just mean what they believe to be right or wrong. Every decent person believes it is wrong to kill someone else except in mortal self-defence. Most people also believe in the Golden Rule: that it is right to treat others as they themselves would like to be treated. Life in any given household will be influenced by beliefs concerning marriage, raising children, how animals should be treated, how to care for the environment, and any strong political views.

People often have strong beliefs on more controversial areas such as same-sex marriage, abortion or military intervention in foreign countries, though they may be more circumspect in expressing these beliefs if they are unsure of their audience. These beliefs will determine how someone responds to an unplanned pregnancy, a colleague's invitation to his or her same-sex wedding, or a son or daughter deciding to join the armed forces.

We are governed by our beliefs in all areas of our lives. These 'headline' examples make this point clear. Things start to get hazier, though, when it comes to pinpointing beliefs about money, health, relationships, career options or personal abilities. This is not because they do not exist, quite the contrary, but your beliefs in these areas of life may be so hard wired into your thinking and behaviours that you may be quite unaware of their presence. So, the task of extracting them from your thoughts for proper examination becomes all the more difficult.

Even if you cannot define all of your beliefs, you are still heavily influenced by them. Someone raised to believe a subtle version of 'money is the root of all evil', after listening to their parents constantly refer to wealthy people as exploitative, will have a tough time trying to succeed as an entrepreneur. A woman, raised with the message that men are smarter and more resilient than women, may rationally dispute this in adult life, but still find it intimidating to have to compete with men in the workplace. So, identified or not, your beliefs pull all your strings.

This filters right down to the minutiae of everyday life. A friend of mine cut her gum on a fish bone as a child and has believed it is a bit dangerous to eat fish ever since, so she has missed out on the delight of seafood her whole life. I believe that checking the pressure in my car tyres in a garage forecourt is a task I cannot manage without getting embarrassingly tangled in the air-hose in public, so I drive around with slightly flat tyres all the time. Beliefs affect everything, large or small.

There is a feedback loop with beliefs and outcomes. If you believe that your colleagues dislike you, you may be hostile towards them. This will make them dislike you and reinforce the belief. Beliefs that generate fear may also expand over time if not challenged. Scary fish get scarier if you are too scared to find out that they are not scary at all. Your beliefs turn your life into a self-fulfilling prophesy. You become what you believe, and you may not even be aware that it is happening.

A Buddhist quote illustrates this principle: "Watch your thoughts; they become words. Watch your words; they become actions. Watch your actions; they become habit. Watch your habits; they become character. Watch your character; it becomes your destiny."

So what has all this got to do with losing weight? Exactly the same principles apply. Someone's beliefs around health, weight, fatness, fitness and food will cascade down into their thinking and behaviours. Stop and consider for a moment what effect the following beliefs might have on everyday life:

- Healthy-living advice is rather earnest and not much fun.
- Once you are very overweight it is impossible to slim down again.
- Exercise is just for slim people.
- Food is my only real luxury in life.

It is easy to see how beliefs like these would undermine any attempt to lose weight. This is precisely why repeat dieters, who have tried every diet under the sun, still struggle to lose weight. The type of diet makes no particular difference. It is the underlying beliefs that determine success or failure. If beliefs change, so will behaviours.

Meanwhile, consider the impact of beliefs that a slim person might typically hold:

- Homemade food tastes much better than convenience food.
- I can eat anything I want, in moderation, without gaining weight.
- Exercise is the most important stress-breaker in my life.
- Luxury is a free afternoon and good book.

The *only* difference between overweight people and thin people is what they believe.

COMMON BELIEFS ABOUT FOOD AND EATING

Having highlighted the central importance of our beliefs, I now want to explore commonly held beliefs relating to health, food and weight in more depth. At this point, I simply want to expose these beliefs rather than try to resolve them. I will discuss strategies that can be used to prepare for a triggering event, and altering beliefs in the next chapter.

The beliefs I discuss below are by no means exhaustive. Your beliefs are highly personal; they make you who you are. No two people are the same. I hope my examples strike a chord with some readers, but I cannot cover all the permutations or intricacies of everyone's beliefs and it would be foolish of me to try. I hope, though, that my examples will encourage you to think about your own beliefs in these areas.

You may have noticed that I have avoided making any reference to feelings or emotions throughout this discussion. Emotions are an enormously important part of life but, like thoughts, they arise from our underlying beliefs. For example, if you believe that spiders are a horrifying and grotesque threat, you will experience revulsion and extreme fear when you find one in the bath. It is the irrational belief that is at fault here, but, given its power, your emotional reaction is appropriate.

Your emotional reactions to the discussion below may help you detect some of your own underlying beliefs, but it is important not to confuse feelings with beliefs. Crucially, there is nothing to be gained by trawling over old grievances and stoking up feelings of recrimination or anger. This would be to miss the point entirely.

Food and Love

The beliefs formed in childhood can exert a lot of power throughout your life. The ways in which food was dealt with within your original family are likely to be the source of core beliefs about food right into adulthood.

Many people believe there is an association between food, nurturance and love. Feeding a child well is one of the most dominant responsibilities of parenting. The instinct to feed a new infant is overwhelming for most new mothers and is integral to forming a bond of love and protectiveness towards the child. Powerful stuff. Fathers, of course, are driven to feed and protect their children too. I emphasise mothering simply because of the sheer physicality of giving birth, breastfeeding and the strong hormonal drives women experience at this time. It forges tight associations between feeding, nurturing, love and being a good mother.

Young children absorb the connection between feeding and mother-love. How that connection is reinforced, loosened or even severed as they get older, however, will set the template for their relationship to food for the rest of their lives. Parents who express their love for their children principally through food, risk overfeeding them. This risk rises if a well-fed child is thought to be highest proof of devoted parenting. Such children are likely to grow up believing that food and love are so closely entwined as to be almost the same thing. Being denied food is experienced as a deprivation of love right into adulthood. By extension, self-compassion may be expressed through food, so there is a tendency to overeat.

Family patterns are often repeated through the generations. People raised to associate love with food will probably replicate this as adults, by providing excess food for others as an expression of their love. Having offerings of food refused may feel like rejection, and food may be pushed at others in order to avoid this.

To the other extreme, if parents withheld food as punishment for misbehaviour, or applied very strict rules about what could or could not be eaten, an association between food and authoritarian control may be created. Children may grow up believing they can gain their parents' approval by complying with these restricted eating habits. On the other hand, they may believe the only way to reclaim control and rebel against parental authority is to overeat. As adults, this belief may morph into a rebellion against anyone trying to dictate what should or should not be eaten, so public health campaigns about good diet, or weight-loss advice from a dietician may be cold-shouldered. There may be a lurking belief that non-compliance is a stand for personal liberty and a snub to authority, so the overeating continues.

Parents who take a more relaxed approach and focus on raising healthy children, rather than simply well-fed children, are far more likely to pass on good attitudes towards food. These parents understand that providing good food for their children is a fundamental parental responsibility, but they do not confuse this with love. Tenderness and affection are expressed in many other ways that have nothing to do with food. Similarly, parents have to set boundaries for their children's behaviour, but this need not be linked to food either.

It is easy to see that someone raised with uncomplicated beliefs about food will be able to enjoy food for its own sake, without hidden or ulterior motives. They are free to be guided by nothing more than their natural hunger and natural satiety; food is just enjoyable fuel to get them through the day. Such easy-going attitudes enables someone to accept the latest health messages without feeling they are bowing to authority. They will have a strong sense of personal sovereignty over food that is confident and relaxed.

Love is love. Food is food. There is no real connection between the two at all. Love, including self-love and self-comforting, does not need food for its expression.

Food as Reward or Treat

Another strong association that many people make is between food and deserving a reward or treat. 'Treat' food tends to be energy-dense fast-food or snacks. The seeds of this are often sown in childhood as well. Most parents bribe their kids with food on the odd occasion for the sake of peace, and it's not a big deal. If this becomes the everyday way to persuade children to complete difficult tasks, though, it may create the belief that getting through any difficult challenge deserves a reward, in particular a food reward. It is not unlike training a pet.

Transplanted into adult life, this belief may convince someone they deserve a bout of overeating, perhaps with some alcohol, because they have had a tough day at work, or an exhausting day with small children who are now finally asleep in their beds. A particular trip-wire for the dieter may be the feeling that a treat is due after struggling through a week of disciplined, low-calorie eating. Ironically, there may be a quite a pronounced sense of injustice if no treat is forthcoming, even though they themselves are withholding it.

As I will explain in the next chapter, it is important to name beliefs. It brings them into focus so they can be properly explored. The belief in the scenario above is: "I believe the negative experience of stress can be reduced by the positive experience of overeating treat food (plus or minus alcohol)." Clearly, this isn't quite right though. It is like trying to treat stress with 'retail therapy' by buying an expensive outfit. It may bring a few moments of cheer, but, when this fades, you go back to same amount of stress you had before, just wearing a new outfit. It doesn't work. Clothes can't treat stress. Neither can pizza or chocolate. You go back to the same amount of stress you had before, just a little fatter. The belief is generating the wrong solution.

There are other consequences of this illogical belief. Firstly, the stress itself goes unaddressed. It is hard work finding solutions to stress; if it were easy, the stress probably wouldn't exist in the first place. This is a Catch-22. If you are already stressed by a tough day, the last thing you may be able to face is the additional stress of looking at the reasons why. It is much easier to push it all away, and reward yourself for just getting through it with some compensatory overeating.

Secondly, the extra food, with or without alcohol, will make you feel worse. The initial fun of indulgence is quickly replaced by feeling guilty, bloated and hung over. You will still be overweight, or gaining more weight. None of it makes sense. Our lives can be full of stress and tough challenges at times. Stress is stress. Food is food. Overeating is the wrong solution to stress.

Food at Celebrations or on Holiday

A common strategy of weight-loss maintainers is that they did not stray from their new dietary regime, even on holidays or during family celebrations. This may seem like remarkable self-control, but in fact their new way of thinking simply uncoupled the association between these special occasions and eating with abandon. Food does tend to be an integral part of celebratory occasions; we have been breaking bread together since prehistoric times. It is not eating on these occasions that is the problem, but overeating. The faulty belief is: "Celebration means being able to eat without limit," or "The only way to really enjoy yourself is to eat freely." You might want to add in: "..plus consume a lot of alcohol," if that applies to you too. No one can sensibly look at such a belief without seeing it is illogical; of course it is possible to have fun and to celebrate without overeating.

63

Observe slim people at these events. Most will relish the good food and will happily take their portion of it, but without overeating. At a large buffet table, laden with delicious food, a slim person will typically want to try a little bit of everything; they will take extra small portions so they have the stomach room to do this. This is the triumph of taste and sensual pleasure over volume for volume's sake. Any celebration is first and foremost about the good company, the shared affection, the stories and the laughter of family and friends, and not the food, pleasurable though this is. Many people also wish to avoid the slightly sedating effect of overeating, so that they can fully enjoy the party.

Holidays are associated with freedom from the normal restrictions of work and home life. This can easily include freedom from food restrictions too, especially if there has been a pre-holiday diet. One of the best things about visiting a foreign country is the opportunity to sample the local cuisine, but it is still possible to do this without overindulging. The problem belief here is: "A good holiday means freedom from all restrictions," or "Freedom includes unlimited eating." This is overeating masquerading as freedom. There is no freedom in compulsive eating.

Plainly, you are just as free not to overeat. You are free to take the same approach as most slim people and place taste above volume by eating a little of everything. Eat small to taste large, and avoid gaining weight into the bargain. Real freedom lies in knowing that you call all the shots in your relationship with food, wherever you are or whatever you are doing. There is no need to be enslaved by a belief that says overeating on holiday or at special events is inevitable or compulsory.

The Problem with Glamour

In the last chapter, I identified a set of pernicious beliefs about body image that the advertising industry plies us with in order to persuade us that there is something wrong if we don't look like the beautiful people in their pictures. Buy their products, they seem to say, and you will be one step closer.

Advertisers create associations with luxury products to fabricate the myth of a world that is glamorous. We are asked to accept their definition of 'cool': graceful, laid-back, knowing and stylish, with sexual tension smouldering just under the surface. This world does not actually exist, however. You could attain the perfect physique, perfect youthfulness, all the right clothes, the best jewellery and go to all the cool places and you still would not find it. The cool places are, in the cold light, just ordinary places full of ordinary people. This is why trying to be glamorous is so elusive, why it always seems to be just out of reach, like a shimmering mirage. Glamour is just a clever illusion that has been manufactured by advertising and celebrity culture. It doesn't mean anything. Yet we buy the products because we buy into the illusion.

What has this got to do with losing weight? It has to do with the misery that fills the gap between self-image and the images of extreme perfection that saturate our world. It has to do with setting unrealistic cosmetic targets, and being dissatisfied with the results because you don't look like a teenage model. Most of all, it is about being manipulated into believing the lie that you are not alright as you are. Our lives are contaminated by these impossible fantasies.

Do not misunderstand me; I am not anti-materialist. It is nice to have nice stuff, and it is fun to dress up occasionally. But you have to lay claim to the aesthetic in your own life, not have this dictated to you by someone else. This means that you alone determine what is or is not beautiful, by your own judgement. Your health, your body, what you choose to wear, how you create your home, the places you visit, the things you engage with, the things you produce, are all on your own terms. This, then, becomes an expression of who you really are, not who or what the advertising industry, the magazines, or anyone else, say you ought to be.

Women and Cookery

The workplace has changed dramatically for women over the past 50 years. Women are as educated as men and, in theory at least, have the same earning power. Reliable birth control, and the feminist movement of the 1970s and 80s, saw more and more women not just entering the professions but increasingly gaining senior positions within them. These were the "women can have it all" years, before post-feminist exhaustion forced them towards something more realistic and flexible.

Back then, many women, especially professional women, formed the belief that it was somehow anti-feminist to be a home-maker; they were not going to be chained to the kitchen sink like their unliberated mothers. It became a badge of honour to be unable to boil an egg or chop an onion because they were too busy building their careers.

Things have eased up a bit nowadays, not least because cooking has been rehabilitated by the rise in popularity of celebrity chefs. Nevertheless, some women still cling to this prejudice against cooking. It demonstrates the way two very different things – professional status and cookery – can become linked in the mind to form a belief: "Learning to cook relegates me to the role of domestic drudge, and undermines my image as a professional woman." As a result, there may be active resistance to learning this vital skill. It also means accepting a long-term diet of convenience food, both inside and outside the home (unless someone else is doing the cooking, of course). It does not necessarily follow that this will make someone overweight, but it increases the likelihood, and will make it much more difficult to lose weight.

Men, Cookery and Health

To this day, less surprise is expressed when a man is unable to cook than a woman. It shows that our society still adheres to rather conventional ideas about gender. Men who were raised in traditional homes, where their mothers did all the cooking and housework, may continue to believe that cookery is really a woman's job. This may segue into other problematic beliefs: "I don't have to think about what I eat because my wife deals with all the food," or "I don't need to learn to cook because one day my future wife will do this."

UK census figures from the last four decades show that more and more people are living alone (about one third of all households are single-person occupied in 2011). More men than women live alone, especially in middle-age. This is a reflection of high divorce rates, and possibly that fewer people get married these days. The average age at first marriage is also rising. Figures from the UK Office for National Statistics in 2011, show that this is currently 31 years for men and 29 years for women, though many couples live together beforehand.[59] The default for anyone who lives alone and cannot cook is to eat processed convenience foods. Men, who believe this is a temporary state of affairs until a domestic goddess appears to provide a stream of home-cooked food "just like mum", need to rethink. They may, in any case, fall in love with a high-flying professional with an aversion to cooking. Besides, women today quite rightly expect men to accept their fair share of domestic responsibilities.

Other erroneous beliefs may coil around this issue: "My wife has greater responsibility for my health than I have," or, more bizarrely, "My future wife will have greater responsibility for my health than me, even though I haven't actually met her yet." Such beliefs encourage men to absolve themselves of responsibility for their own health, and obviously there is a problem with that. More painful beliefs may run in tandem with this if a single man believes that learning to cook is tantamount to admitting he may always be alone. Clearly it means no such thing; indeed, it would likely improve his chances of impressing a woman.

I am not suggesting for a minute that this applies to all men. I know plenty of men who are good cooks, and are rightly proud of this skill. Fortunately, the recent spate of alpha male chefs appearing on our television screens have more or less killed off any notion that cooking is effeminate, even when they are preparing delicate confectionery. It is a trend increasingly taken up by younger men.

It is delightful to be able to cook. Preparing a meal can be surprisingly therapeutic after a long day. Dismissing this as a chore is a state of mind. Cooks get absorbed in the whole process of trying new recipes, and tracking down the best ingredients. The inevitable boost to health is a huge bonus. It is no accident that men and women who can cook tend to be leaner and healthier than those who cannot. Go figure.

Food Wastage

Not wasting food is sensible, thrifty and good for the environment. Without doubt, the best way to do this is to avoid buying surplus food in the first place. This means meal planning and smart shopping. A mismatch of food, purchased in high volume with a lower turnover of food in the home, means that spare food will inevitably reach its sell-by date before it is consumed. In addition, there are usually some spare food scraps during cooking, and leftovers if too much food was prepared in the first place.

Most households have at least some food wastage. It does not really matter from which point in the food cycle surplus food arises, what matters is how it is dealt with. Few people would take issue with the belief that it is wrong to waste food. The word 'waste', however, conjures up the image of a bin, so the belief shifts to: "It is wrong to put food in the bin." The corollary of this belief is: "Surplus food is not wasted as long as it is eaten."

In response to this belief, surplus food on the point of expiring may get eaten, in addition to the day's meals; spare food may be grazed during cooking, rather than being discarded or stored; there may be insistence on plate-clearing at mealtimes; or mouthfuls of leftovers eaten before plates are scraped. If you are overweight, though, this surplus food has already been wasted whether you eat it or not. It does not matter if it is thrown into the bin or thrown onto your thighs, so it might as well go in the bin. The issue is one of location, not thrift. Seeing a lot of food go into the bin may, in any case, encourage more prudent shopping habits, which is where true thrift lies.

Food and Assertiveness

In the previous chapter, I mentioned a study which found that people who were confident enough to refuse food that was offered to them had a better chance of successfully losing weight than those who found this difficult.[60] I should be clear that this does not mean giving in to temptation. I am referring to accepting food that you would rather refuse because you find it uncomfortable to say no. This can be hard to do if the person pushing food at you seems to be threatening a bit of a sulk if you do not accept. Subtle manipulations may used to force your hand, such as being told the food was specially selected or prepared for you, and that this took much time. As mentioned above, some people associate food with love and may take a refusal of their food as a personal rejection.

Overeating can also be an isolating experience for someone who is overweight or obese. They may try to suppress feelings of loneliness by encouraging others to overeat too. If you suspect food is being pushed at you for this reason, saying no may feel like you are refusing to offer solace or solidarity.

In both of the above scenarios, the underlying belief is: "I will create conflict that I cannot handle if I refuse this food." But these problems do not belong to you, they belong to the person pushing the food at you. Taking the food will not change this, so you might as well stand your ground and say no. It is also straightforwardly possible to decline food graciously in a way that undermines any justification for a sulk. There are other ways to reassure someone of your affection, and better ways to cheer up someone who is feeling a bit downhearted and lonely.

When someone makes a major life change it often has an impact on others. If snack foods and soda drinks have always been readily available at home, family members may feel aggrieved if this suddenly changes. It is a bit tough for someone who is working towards a healthy weight to have a lot of these foods around, though, so this needs to be addressed. Someone who fears conflict, however, may be deterred from doing this. The belief here is: "Keeping the peace is more important than my health." I hope anyone holding such a belief will stop to consider its serious implications. The dynamics of every family are different, but people can be surprisingly supportive when they are presented with a strong case for change. Health is always a strong case.

Denial of Weight Gain from Overeating

I have so far concentrated on beliefs that are based on associations between things that have no actual connection, such as love and food, or gender and cookery. Some beliefs do the opposite and break the link between things that are absolutely connected. This is the strange phenomenon of denial and it is powerful. The odd thing about denial is that the factual connection between things is generally accepted; it is acknowledged that overeating causes fatness, for example. In spite of knowing this, however, some people who are overweight do not acknowledge that their overeating causes their fatness. Indeed, many deny they overeat at all. The root cause of such a denial will be unique to that person, but the problem may seem so overwhelming that the only solution is to suppress it.

It is much easier to deny the detrimental day-to-day effects of any habit, such as smoking, when these are incrementally so small they are hidden from view. A smoker cannot see the small tumour in his lungs being drip-fed carcinogens every time he takes in a lungful of smoke, so he carries on smoking. We cannot see high blood pressure, or tightening arteries, or cells starting to resist insulin, so we carry on engaging in health-damaging behaviours in blissful denial.

There is a similar version of this drip-drip effect that mutes the connection between overeating and gaining weight. A meal of excessive calories will become a fresh layer of fat across the body within a few hours of consumption, but this new flesh is spread evenly over the whole body, so it cannot be seen. Nor can the skin be felt stretching a little to accommodate this new flesh, though this is exactly what is happening. A slim person who puts on a few pounds over a week or two will notice their clothing is tighter, and be alerted to the weight gain. Someone who is overweight or obese may not notice the same weight gain because it is spread over a larger surface area. It may be further concealed if loose clothing is worn. As the weight gain is proportionately smaller, and therefore more invisible, it may seem like an inconsequential drop in the ocean. The cumulative effects of meals like this can be more easily dismissed, until the day of reckoning on the weighing scales.

The belief can be identified easily: "I am already so overweight that this calorie-laden meal won't make that much difference." The same belief will accommodate frequent snacks. The trouble is, if this rationale is used constantly to justify such overeating, then, quite obviously, it will make a huge difference.

The same disconnect applies to other behaviours where immediate effects are invisible. Nearly everyone knows that a moderate diet full of fresh vegetables and fruit is more nourishing than a diet of junk food, yet many people are sceptical about how much difference it would really make to how they feel. One effect of a chronically poor diet is that it will have made someone feel below par for so long that they will have come to accept this as normal. But the high-nutrient content of good food is rapidly shifted into the body's cells, in much the same way that fat is after a high-calorie meal. Within a week or so, the difference will be tangible as more energy and better mood; within a month eyes and skin will be clearer and weight may have dipped. These effects on the body are real. It is like putting high-grade petrol into a car. You notice the difference in performance.

All the scenarios above are simplifications. I cannot cover all the angles of our complex relationship with food. Perhaps none of these scenarios apply to you; perhaps all of them do. What matters is that you start to think about your own beliefs about food, even if they feel like 'truths' for the time being.

HOLDING CONTRADICTORY BELIEFS SIMULTANEOUSLY

Sometimes one's own behaviour can be a mystery. You may have an important report to write for a fast-approaching deadline, but find yourself doing battle with your procrastination. You may want a promotion, but avoid applying for it when the opportunity arises. You may want a child, but keep on using contraception. You may want to lose weight, but keep on overeating. These contradictions arise when we hold two opposing beliefs at the same time. Psychotherapists call this 'cognitive dissonance', and it is very common. Generally, such conflicting beliefs are hidden from conscious view, but, like all beliefs, they govern your thoughts and behaviours, so you end up in an apparently inexplicable tug-of-war with yourself. The following examples may help to clarify how this can happen.

Steve, who is in his 30s, has worked for the same company for ten years. He knows he should have climbed the career ladder by now, but he has avoided promotion when more senior positions became available. The first time he thought he was too inexperienced; the second time, he and his wife had a new baby and he wanted to concentrate on his home life. Now another senior post has become vacant and Steve has run out of excuses. He knows the job better than anyone, and the extra money would help the family finances, but although he is respected by his co-workers, he cannot imagine having to supervise them, or pull someone up for poor work. He dreads the responsibility and the risk of conflict. Steve is being pulled in different directions by two opposite beliefs. The first is: "I will fail and be exposed as a fraud, because none of my co-workers will take me seriously as a manager." The second is: "After this length of time, I have to apply for promotion to protect my professional credibility." Until Steve acknowledges this internal conflict, and addresses his fears, he will continue to sway back and forth between these two positions. He will be stuck between them.

Grace, also in her 30s, did a lot of travelling with her friends in her early twenties. It was the happiest time of her life. She yearns to travel again and spends a lot of time pouring over brochures. Her career has flourished over the years but now all her friends are married with children, and she has no one to go travelling with anymore. The thought of travelling alone fills her with trepidation. Grace is also being pulled in opposite directions by her beliefs. She believes that travelling is the best way to live life to the full, but she also believes it is dangerous for a woman to travel alone, and that there is no point in travelling if there is no one to share it with. Grace will continue to deny herself the joy of travelling while this internal conflict goes unresolved.

Superficially, the conflict at the heart of trying to lose weight may seem more obvious than either of the examples above: you have to eat less to achieve the desired weight loss but you get hungry and want food. But it is far more complicated than this. A lot of people believe that losing weight will solve many problems in their lives, not just their weight problem. For example, they believe it will revive a lacklustre relationship, improve their career prospects, or give them the confidence to stand up to people who put them down. A contrary belief undermines all this: "Life without the pleasure of abundant food is a depressing prospect." None of this is true, of course, but it is easy to see how it forms a loop of self-sabotage.

In his book *The Path of Least Resistance*, Robert Fritz discusses this phenomenon with regard to creative blocks, but it works just as well for the dilemma around losing weight and overeating.[61] Fritz outlines what he calls 'structural tension' to describe this internal tug-of-war. He pictures the afflicted person tethered by two pieces of elastic, pulling them in the opposite directions of their conflicting beliefs. At the midpoint, the elastic on either side has equal tension. As the person moves toward the goals of one belief, the elastic tension on the opposite side increases and starts to exert a forceful pull. Eventually, this pull will be too strong for the person to resist and they will recoil, not just back to the midpoint, but beyond it. This will then create tension on the other side, and the whole thing starts again. The person bounces back and forth between the two beliefs in a pattern Fritz calls oscillation.

Fritz' model, applied to weight and overeating, finds the overweight, food-loving person standing between the desire to lose weight and the desire for their favourite foods. By applying will power, he or she may soldier towards the goal of weight loss, despite the increasing counter-tension pulling them back towards the rich food. When this tension gets high, even a small relaxation of effort will allow the taut elastic to spring them back, past the midpoint, and force surrender to their desire for the food. This may even be marked with episodes of binge eating that seem hard to control. Meanwhile, tension has now been created on the opposite 'need-to-lose-weight' side of the balance. This is experienced first as guilt and frustration, but, as overeating continues, gradually builds up into despair and self-loathing. When this clips panic, the person is yanked back onto a dieting regime and the whole thing starts all over again. It is worth noting, that the recoil back onto a dieting regime is very often a treatment for the panic, rather than the excess weight. This is why crank, rapid weight-loss diets are so commercially successful.

So, if this applies to you, how do you break free? Fritz argues that it is not possible to break these counter tensions from within the system. You have to step out of the structure and start afresh. This means identifying these opposing beliefs and challenging them. It may be possible to break one obstructive belief in order to release the power of the other. Alternatively, both beliefs may need to be dismantled. You must end up with only one dominant belief, one main goal pulling you in one clear direction. Fritz calls this the path of least resistance.

Even when they are illogical or self-sabotaging, your beliefs have the power to dictate outcomes in your life. You become what you believe. I have worked through a lot of different scenarios in order to demonstrate this. Beliefs masquerade as truths. Understanding this creates room for manoeuvre. If you believe that A, B and C are true then your mind will cast them in stone and never challenge them. If, on the other hand, you accept that you just believe A, B and C to be the case at this time, you embrace a degree of flexibility in your thinking that opens the door for change.

Triggering events, or epiphanies, change core beliefs so completely that it becomes impossible to revert back to the old way of doing things; they have life-altering power. But what if you have not experienced a triggering event? What if you think you had one, but it did not seem to last? Is there some way to initiate your own, long lasting triggering event? I wholeheartedly believe there is, for the simple reason that I have done this successfully in my own life, and witnessed others do the same. In the following chapter, I discuss the necessary steps to bring this about.

Preparing for Your Own Triggering Event

I hope I have convinced you of the importance of holding life-enhancing beliefs, and freeing yourself from the ones that are obstructive, or even damaging. Beliefs are tenacious. They cling on, even if the original events that created them took place a long ago, and despite growing evidence against them. When the weight of evidence becomes too strong, however, a belief will break under the strain, and be replaced with something new. This moment may seem sudden, and will cause an immediate shift in perspective – a triggering event. In most cases, the mind has actually been preparing for this event for some time, often just barely within conscious thought. Although the mind usually does this instinctively, it is possible to actively prepare for it. You can do the groundwork and set yourself up for your own triggering event, even though you cannot know beforehand what this event will be.

In this chapter, I describe the steps needed to identify and challenge incorrect beliefs which may be affecting your health and weight. This takes time. Anyone who thinks they can change their beliefs in the space of reading one book needs to set more realistic expectations. Knee-jerk reactions are understandable, but they will stop you from seeing how your beliefs are influencing your behaviour. This process needs patience, so you can make proper observations.

Some say it is only possible to change core beliefs with the help of a psychotherapist. I do not agree but with an important caveat. This process does need a period of reflection; it might mean looking at some difficult things in your life. We all have problems we would prefer not to think about, but this makes it hard to see obstructing beliefs. Healthy adults are perfectly capable of examining the workings of their own psyche, without the help of a counsellor or therapist, but this simple picture changes where someone has faced extreme difficulties in the past. For example, if someone has a history of a violent childhood, post-traumatic-stress disorder, or fragile mental health, especially if this continues to have an impact on their life, then seeking the help of a professional therapist is likely to be of considerable benefit.

Surprisingly few people examine their own beliefs. If something is clearly wrong with the picture of your life, however, particularly if this has been the case for a long time, then your underlying beliefs are probably tripping you up. One particular difficulty is that beliefs cannot always be distinguished from truth: they feel true. But if you hold onto something as a truth, you will not be able to change it. You can change what you believe.

An essential first step in dismantling a belief is to inject it with doubt. From the outset, you must be willing to recast your 'truths' about health and being overweight as beliefs, even if you have to take this on faith for now. By demoting a truth to a belief you weaken its foundations with that first vital crack of doubt for, by default, you have to accept the possibility that the belief might be wrong.

Do not assume all your beliefs are logical. Interestingly, your rational mind often knows when they are not. Consider this: if you know it is incorrect to think that a slim person is more attractive and disciplined than someone who is overweight, but, if you are honest, find that you believe it nonetheless, which one of you knows this is incorrect and which one of you still believes it? Are there two of you? Well, in a way, yes.

This is typically described as the conscious and the subconscious mind. They are distinct but not separate; they normally work together so closely that you feel you are of one mind nearly all of the time. The conscious mind feeds its understanding of the world to the subconscious, which locks the pieces of it into beliefs and instructions for subsequent thoughts and behaviour. This is how we learn from experience.

If we misinterpret experience, or if long-ago experience is no longer relevant to the present, our incorrect or out-of-date beliefs will produce a wrong picture in our lives. The conscious mind can see this, even if it cannot always see the correct solutions. It can, however, start to mount rational challenge to this wrong picture with analysis and questioning. In this way, your conscious mind exerts pressure on subconscious beliefs until they give way. In other words, you can change your beliefs with deliberate effort. This can happen quite quickly, but more often than not it takes time to wear the subconscious mind down to the point where it finally surrenders an obstructing belief.

It is not an easy thing to do, but consider the consequences of giving up before you have properly defeated a defeating belief. It puts you back in the dubious position of waiting for a health crisis, and no one wants that. It also takes you back to square one trying diet after diet, pitting yourself against powerful obstructing beliefs that will drag you back to failure time and again. It is like constantly trying to swim upstream and it's exhausting. I would argue, that it is so exhausting it is not worth putting yourself through the trauma of another dieting battle until you have the backing of solid, life-enhancing beliefs. These are the sine qua non (without this, nothing) of major life change, and they will carry you downstream beautifully.

SOMETHING WRONG WITH THE PICTURE OF YOUR LIFE

You would not be reading this book if you did not already know there was something wrong with the picture of your life, though you may think it is only because you are overweight. Many people are baffled by how they came to be overweight in the first place, especially if they need to lose a lot of weight. They may be even more baffled about why they have found it so difficult to correct this. The different areas of our lives are always interlinked, however, so a wider look at life becomes essential in order to see the picture accurately. This matters because becoming overweight does not happen in isolation from the rest of your life.

It is time to do some detective work. It is time to take stock of your whole life, not just stock of your health and weight. This is like taking a series of snapshots of your life and laying them out on a table. Importantly, these are snapshots of your present life, and not of your past. If it helps, imagine you are someone else looking in at your life from the sidelines. What would they see? This might be unsettling, especially if there is emotional turbulence in your life, but try not to be distracted by strong feelings if you can manage it. It is particularly important not to waste time on feelings of bitterness or anger towards others. You must be at the centre of this picture, no one else. Above all, do not blame yourself if there are things in your life you are unhappy about. Also, at this point, do not look for solutions to the problems you find. Just try to see the picture as clearly as you can.

If you are like most people, your life will be a mixed bag. For example, you may be pretty content in your home life but miserable at work, or vice versa. Perhaps you have a great social life but struggle with debts. Perhaps you have what could be the perfect life, except you work such long hours you never get to enjoy it, or you have no one special to share it with. We are all different.

Although all areas of life overlap, reviewing the overall landscape of your life might be easier if you compartmentalise it, and take a separate snapshot of each area in your mind's eye. Take mental pictures of the following areas in your life, but not the areas of health and weight for now:

- your relationship status
- family situation
- extended family situation
- your home
- work within the home (housework)
- financial situation
- work outside the home
- friendships
- social life
- leisure time
- the overall pace of life
- your main skills
- the direction of your life as you see it at present

Feel free to add any other areas that apply to you that I have not included.

It is important to give yourself enough time to do this, although, as you think through the list, each picture will probably come to mind pretty quickly. It is entirely up to you how you do this. You may find it helpful to write it all down under separate headings, or even draw up a table. I recommend this because it is easier to keep track. But you may prefer to mull it over while soaking in a hot bath, or going for a long, quiet walk. Do whatever works for you, as long as you remember to assess your life as it is now, and avoid blaming yourself or others if what you see is less than perfect.

As your mind looks at each of these pictures, you will instinctively label them along the lines of: wonderful, good, OK, non-existent, bothersome, vexing. Choose any labels you want, but avoid extreme labels, such as 'total nightmare', or 'absolute chaos', because these are highly emotional and it is important to try to contain strong emotions while you do this exercise, if you can. You need to take a dispassionate view in order to see these pictures accurately.

What you should end up with is the unique landscape of your own life. It should give you a more focused picture of the areas in your life that are happy, content and stable (not to be confused with perfect), and those that are not. With this whole-life view in front of you, I want you to consider the final category of health, but first I want you to be clear about what this means.

Health is a unifying term covering different things that contribute to or undermine wellness. It includes:

- physical ailments and disabilities
- general fitness
- mental stability
- sleep pattern
- eating pattern
- diet

- weight

- physical activity

- sexual health

- relationships with alcohol, drugs or tobacco.

Using these pointers, take a mental snapshot of your own health as it is today. Write it down if you wish. When you have a clear picture, hold it up against the landscape of your life and see how your health relates to each of its territories. It is worth being quite systematic about this, in order to see how your health affects, and is affected by, each area in your life. These are the links you want to pin down; this is the point of the exercise. Health and weight cannot be carved out as issues to be dealt with in isolation from the rest of your life, and this must be accepted if long term solutions to health problems are to be found.

For example, you may see links between financial difficulties and poor sleep, or between a sparse social life and overeating, or between long working hours and a lack of physical activity. The following examples may help.

MICHAEL, 36 YEARS OLD

Michael works as a senior manager at an IT company. He is well paid but works long hours. He lives on his own in a large city-centre apartment, which is full of all the latest gadgets. He speaks to his mother a couple of times a month by phone, but doesn't see much of his sister who is busy with a young family. He goes to the pub with a couple of old friends from university to watch TV football on Saturday afternoons, but doesn't go out much apart from this. Michael has been single for around six years. He always thought he would be married with a family by this age, but thinks his busy career got in the way.

He has tried internet dating a few times, but he found it a bit of an ordeal.

Michael started putting on weight when he went to university and was 300 lbs by the time he was twenty five. He is known as Big Mike and can drink up to ten pints of beer on Saturdays. He knows he is unfit. He bought some weights and a rowing machine a couple of years ago but cannot remember the last time he used them. When his friends asked him to join them for five-aside football he said he was too busy. The truth is he cannot really run anymore and didn't want to let the team down. He is tired when he gets home from work and just wants to relax in front of his computer with some easy food and a few beers. Although Michael has a good job, he knows the picture of his life is not right. He is lonely. He doesn't get the chance to meet single women very often, and he worries they will be put off by his size anyway. He is not sure where this is all going, mostly he tries not to think about it too much.

MELANIE, 48 YEARS OLD

Melanie works part-time at a supermarket and is married with two teenagers. Her life is hectic. As well as working shifts, she does all the cooking and housework at her home, and at her mother's a few miles away. Like many parents, she also drives her children everywhere; her 17 year old son is a champion swimmer and has to be ferried back and forth to frequent training sessions, and her 18 year old daughter needs to be driven to and from college. Melanie also collects them from their nights out at weekends. She doesn't get the chance to see her own friends much these days, she is just too busy, but she misses their company.

Melanie put on a lot of weight with two pregnancies in quick succession. She tried every diet you could name but never returned to her pre-pregnancy size. She became the classic yo-yo dieter; losing some weight but regaining more over and over again. Finally, she gave up and stopped weighing herself, but when she visited her doctor he insisted. Melanie had become obese; her BMI was 35 kg/m². Her blood pressure was also high and she had to start medication to bring this down. She is so busy looking after other people, however, she is not sure that she has time to think about her own health right now.

Melanie feels she does everything at home, but no one ever thanks her, or offers to help. Her husband only helps if she nags him, so it is just easier to do it all herself. The one thing Melanie sees as compensation for all her hard work is settling in front of the television most evenings with a big spread of food. She knows the food is fattening, but she is already so overweight that a bit more hardly matters. She does plan to sort her health out eventually, when the kids are older, but her life is too stressful to give this up just yet.

KATIE, 24 YEARS OLD

Katie works in an office and lives at home with her parents and two younger brothers. They are all close and have extended family nearby. Every weekend there is a big get-together. Their lives revolve around food and the whole family is overweight. Her parents prepare a huge meal for the five of them every night, followed by snacks in front of the television. Katie also goes out with her friends a couple of nights a week, though her mum scolds her for drinking too much. When she is with her slimmer friends, she feels self-conscious about her weight and tries to compensate by being the party girl. It gets her attention from men, though not the type of man she would prefer.

Katie is just over 200 lbs and has tried to lose weight a couple of times before going on holiday with her friends.

Though she quickly lost 10 lbs each time, she regained more than this soon afterwards. These were crash diets. They horrified her mother, who reassured her about her appearance, and coaxed her into eating again. What Katie really wants is to meet some nice guy to settle down with, so she can start a family of her own. Recently, she has started to wonder if she is fit enough for a young family; she can barely run for a bus. In any case, she doesn't know how to change things without upsetting her family.

It is easy to look at someone else's life and see where the problems lie. It is much harder to be so objective about your own life, but this is the kind of snapshot that brings things into focus. It is what you are aiming for. It can be quite brief but still comprehensive.

What should be clear, from the three examples above, is that there are quite different reasons why Michael, Melanie and Katie are overweight. This is why the standard eat-less-do-more advice rarely works on its own. It does not address broader, underlying issues. It is like a doctor suggesting a treatment without having investigated or diagnosed an illness. The chances of success would be low. If you want to solve a problem, you have to know what the real problem is in the first place.

It may seem obvious that overeating and/or lack of physical activity cause the problem of being overweight, but these are symptoms of something else. It is why this stage of investigation is so important. Having taken a snapshot of your own life, you now have to narrow down your focus, in order to see which territory is at the heart of your own weight problems.

IDENTIFYING RELEVANT LIFE TERRITORIES

After doing the exercise above, you may be able to spot the areas in your life that are contributing to your being overweight quite easily. For example, you may know this is linked to getting promotion and switching from being on your feet all day to working long hours at a desk. For many people, however, identifying the areas in their life that are the cause of their overeating or lack of activity is much trickier. There may be also be confusion between causes and outcomes.

At this stage of the process, you are looking for the areas in your life that are causing or encouraging overeating and/or lack of activity. Do not confuse these with areas in your life that have become a problem because you are overweight. Michael is overweight because of a combination of factors: his work and leisure time are both sedentary; he eats a lot of fast-food and beer because he cannot cook; and his social life revolves around alcohol. But being overweight has *created* problems in other areas of his life: it deters him from participating in sport; and, due to his low confidence, discourages him from seeking a partner. Later on, it will be useful to consider the effects of being overweight, but for now I want you to concentrate on the areas of your life that are contributing to overeating or a lack of activity.

This needs courage. For example, it might not be easy to admit that your home life is not that great, and that overeating is linked to the stress this causes. Or perhaps you wish you had more friends to go out with at weekends, and make up for this by having a lot of food at home on your own. You have to be honest with yourself. I can offer examples, but only you know what the different territories of your life look like.

If you are finding it hard to pin down the specific areas in your life that are associated with overeating or lack of exercise, you may be blocking out something you do not really want to see. If you are feeling stuck, ask yourself what is going on whenever you find yourself overeating. Notice the place, time, who you are with, or not with. What else you are doing? What sort of day you have had? What is happening the following day? Please don't be hard on yourself as you do this. Treat this as important detective work. Make the necessary observations and be glad that you are making progress. Facing up to something that is unsettling is the start of something positive, even if it is a bit frightening at first.

Beware red herrings. I have heard many overweight people say things like: "I am overweight because I just like food too much," or "I am overweight because I have the self-discipline of a child." These self-berating beliefs can be challenged like any others, but they are also smokescreens that hide deeper issues.

Someone like Melanie, above, might have a tough time unpicking what was really going on in her life. Melanie does not like to focus on herself. As an outsider looking in, it is easy to see that her family life is unbalanced, and that there is an uneven distribution of labour within the home. Sitting down to a feast several times a week is Melanie's redress. She believes it is her reward for all her giving, despite the health alarm bells that are starting to ring.

The territory in your life that is linked to overeating or lack of exercise may not be an unhappy one. Gaining weight after getting promotion does not mean getting promotion is a problem, particularly if you enjoy your new role and the bigger salary that comes with it. Other happy areas that might be connected to overeating could be having got married in the last couple of years, or having had a much-wanted baby. You have to be honest if these areas are linked to your being overweight in order to solve this.

Katie's situation falls into this category. She has a very happy family life which is nevertheless, and undeniably, at the heart of her overeating. Katie has no idea what to do about this. There is also the issue of the amount of alcohol she consumes when out with friends, and the amount of food that is eaten on the way home from a night out.

Do not worry if the problems you find seem unsolvable at the moment. You may feel some anxiety rising within you about this, or feel like pushing the problems away in case they make you feel a bit depressed. Remember you are still just investigating; you are still doing the reconnaissance work. You are drawing the overweight/overeating/low-activity map of your life so that you can take a calm look at it. Persist until you are confident you have a pretty accurate map, even if some aspects of it make uncomfortable viewing for now.

CAPTURING AND NAMING YOUR BELIEFS

It is time to take the next step and actually name the beliefs you hold about your health, about being overweight, and about other, relevant areas in your life. Beliefs, especially when they have been held for a long time, can be hard to see; you will probably have to search for them. It needs quiet time and a lot of concentration. When you do see them, you will realise that most of them have been hiding in plain sight. It is like the old saying that fish can't see water.

First, I must say something about how beliefs are named. It is important to get this right, otherwise beliefs get mixed up with emotions, or even excuses, and this will not work. Beliefs are usually expressed as short statements. So, for example: "I believe that exercise is only for slim people," rather than "I don't take formal exercise because I just can't face it." An excuse will not tell you much. The second statement should make you ask why you cannot face exercise. It may be that you cannot face being overweight in a group of slim people, or having to struggle with exercise in public. This is really about dignity. The actual belief is: "I believe that overweight people look clumsy when they exercise." How beliefs are named, and how they are expressed, matters a great deal.

Take each of the areas in your life that contribute to your being overweight in turn and write down everything that you believe about them. A stream-of-consciousness style will serve you well as you do this. Write as freely as you can. Inevitably this will include some things that are very private, so choose a private time and place, and keep your notes somewhere safe. It might be harder to contain your emotions during this exercise. A particular belief may ignite strong feelings, and you might be aware of these before you have discovered the belief itself. Emotions can give you clues about your beliefs; generally speaking the stronger the emotion the closer you are to seeing the belief. You have to keep a cool head at this point in order to see past strong feelings to the belief that is generating them. It means staying put and not taking flight.

Convention has it that you must trawl over your past and your childhood in order to understand yourself and fix your present. I am not so sure. It can be interesting, and sometimes useful, to trace the origins of your beliefs, but it is not a necessary condition of identifying them or changing them. We all carry the stories of our lives around in our heads, even though our memories are notoriously unreliable and one-sided. Prominent narratives from the past may be so dominant that you come to believe they have defined the course of your life, but this is not necessarily so. It is just as likely that more routine or fleeting events created the beliefs in your mind, though these memories may be more concealed. If you single out a belief that is blocking you from moving forward, it does not matter much where it came from. What matters is that you name it correctly now.

A correctly identified belief will strike an immediate chord of recognition within you. This is an important marker, even for a belief that seems quite peculiar in the cold light of day. If this reaction is missing, be suspicious that you have not quite nailed what it is you really believe about something. This striking-of-a-chord sensation should also help you distinguish between what you really believe and what you think you ought to believe, or what you wished you could believe. For example, you may want to believe that everything at home is fine but know, deep down, that this is not really true. You may then feel a pang of recognition when you admit that you overeat in response to the stress at home.

I cannot identify your beliefs; you are the only person who can do that. I can only provide examples. Here are the beliefs Michael, Melanie and Katie identified as they did this exercise.

MICHAEL

Michael identified his long working hours, his sedentary lifestyle, his poor knowledge about food and his social life as the factors in his life that were contributing to his weight problem. The beliefs he wrote down were:

- I believe that I do not have time to improve my health.

- I believe that playing on my computer with a big meal and a few beers helps me unwind after a stressful day at work.

- I believe that there is no point in cooking when I can buy my favourite convenience foods online.

- I believe that healthy food is boring rabbit food and not enough for a big guy like me.

- I believe that Saturdays at the pub would be no fun at all without the beer.

When Michael thought more deeply, however, he tracked down beliefs that he had not been fully aware of before:

- I believe that I command people's attention at work because I am a big guy.

- I believe that a lovely woman will just appear from somewhere, and put my life right.

- I believe that the health problems that affect people who are overweight don't apply to me because I'm only 36.

It may be tempting to read this list as though they are statements of fact, but they are not. While it is true that Michael holds these beliefs, none of them are actually true. It is easy to see, though, how they have shaped his life. It is also easy to see that his aching hope that things will magically improve of their own accord is wrong. These beliefs have locked Michael into this life.

MELANIE

Melanie knew perfectly well that her evenings of overeating were compensation for her exhausting home life, but it needed courage to look at why home life had become so exhausting in the first place. She felt like she was opening a can of worms. These are the beliefs she wrote down:

- I believe that my spreads of food are a reward for all my hard work. I deserve this.

- I believe that I devote nearly all my time to the needs of my family. My food treats are the only thing I have for myself.

- I believe that my family would fall apart if I didn't keep on top of everything.

- I believe that my family's needs are more important than my health.

- I believe that I will address my weight problem when the children are older.

This made Melanie feel quite angry towards her family. She felt indignant that they took her for granted. It helped her to see more painful beliefs:

- I believe that all the work I do at home makes me seem indispensable.

- I believe that my children are growing up and won't need me for much longer.

Like Michael, Melanie thought she was just describing the truth of her life as she listed her beliefs. It was a tough exercise because it forced her to see that the reasons she overate were more complex and frightening than she had admitted before. She was quite disturbed by this, because she could not see how any of it could be solved.

KATIE

Katie had a different set of beliefs. She wrote:

- I believe that family life is all about food.

- I believe that none of us know how to eat any other way.

- I believe that it is not possible for me to eat differently from my family.

- I believe that I will upset my parents if I refuse their food.

- I believe that we shelter each other from the fat-shaming and jibes from the outside world because we are all overweight together.

- I believe my family will think I am criticising them if I lose weight.

It was insightful and honest of Katie to identify these beliefs. She did not know how to change her situation, and wondered if it was all a bit hopeless. But Katie was finding it harder to ignore the consequences of being so overweight, and the tension between this and her family life were starting to get her down.

Some people will be tempted to turn away at this point, and find an easier way of dealing with their weight problem. There isn't one. Perhaps your hope for a simple solution seems more complicated now that you have stepped back to see the other factors in your life that are involved. Trying to get hold of what you believe about something can be like trying to catch a greased pig in a dark room, but it is worth the effort. Without knowing what you believe there is no way forward. You will simply revert to another version of the old way, and you already know that does not work.

THE DESIRE FOR CHANGE

It may seem strange to ask you how much you want to change things, given that you are reading this book in the first place. Surely, it is obvious that you do. People who are utterly fed up with being overweight may feel their desire to change this is so strong the question barely needs asking. The question I actually ask you, however, is this: if your desire to lose weight is so strong, why has it not already won the day? What more powerful desire is blocking its path? The desire to change is central to success in any venture. The critical issue is whether or not the strength of this desire is greater than the desire to protect the status quo.

Long term weight loss needs a permanent change in lifestyle; it does means eating less and being more active. There is no sensible path to losing weight without this, and there is no magic wand. The sought-after desire is that these activities themselves should become straightforward and sustainable. As you think about implementing them within your own life, however, your beliefs will start to fight you. Take a moment to imagine foregoing the big portions of food, the snacks, the excess alcohol, as well as greatly increasing your level of activity. Imagine doing this forever. You may only have a shaky hope you can pull this off, even though you never have before. What is it that fills the vacuum left by the excess food? What is it that stands in your way when you think of all that exercise? Whatever it is, it will give rise to feelings of dread.

It is the dread you need to get hold of. This is your subconscious taking all your obstructing beliefs and putting bells and whistles on them to sound the alarm. It is telling you it is much easier and safer to change nothing. You have its full attention. That is why I am using the word 'dread', and not some softer word, such as 'resistance'. Your subconscious cannot ignore dread.

In your mind, I want you to walk right into the middle of the dread. I want you to stand there and stare it in the face, and I want you to name the belief that supports it. Find the words, even if you need a few tries to find the words that are just right. Whatever it is that you dread when you think about a lifetime of eating less, drinking less, and doing more exercise is *exactly* what is stopping you from losing weight and maintaining this.

Read that again; it is the most important sentence in the whole book.

Knowing what this dread is, so explicitly, can feel like a punch in the stomach but it is a massive step forward. This dread will be at the heart of the central belief that is holding you back. The desire to protect yourself from this dread has, so far, been stronger than your desire to permanently change your lifestyle. Awareness of this is the first big step in preparing your mind for the triggering event that will break the belief, dissolve the dread and set you free.

Once you have named the central belief that incurs this dread, carry it, and the beliefs you named earlier, around with you for a while. Do this for up to a week or two if need be. Get to know them well but constantly remind yourself that they are just beliefs, not truths. See how they influence your thinking and affect your behaviour. I am serious when I say you should not try to solve any problems just yet. Just make observations of them.

It is human instinct to try to solve problems quickly. You may be tempted to come up with an immediate plan, any plan, even a slightly crazy plan, because this seems more bearable than having to live with the uncertainty of an unsolved problem. Implementing short-term solutions, however, will distract you from the more important task of becoming familiar with the deep beliefs that are holding you back. Quick solutions conceal the real stumbling blocks; they solve nothing in the long run.

MICHAEL

Michael knew that he would have to change if he wanted his life to change. He had hoped that his future wife would just appear in his life somehow, out of the blue, without him actually having to do anything to bring this about. He has been holding out for this for several years, however, and nothing had changed. In fact his weight problem and his loneliness were getting worse.

Looking through his list of beliefs made Michael feel even more stuck, but he acknowledged that he was at least looking at the issues, which was progress of a sort. Michael would have given a lot to get back to the 160 lb weight he was when he was eighteen, before all the partying and beer drinking at university took over. When he imagined a life without his big fast-food meals and all the beer, however, he realised it would mean facing life outside of work completely sober.

Michael is not an alcoholic but he was still shocked by this admission. It forced him to see how much he dreaded having to face the emptiness of his life when he should have been in his prime. The sense of dread was heightened when he admitted to himself that he had no idea how to fix this. The computer games, the fast-food and the beers reminded him of his younger years at university when he was part of a big social group. Continuing with this made him feel like he was still one of the guys. It blotted out the one deep-down belief that he had been avoiding: "I believe that none of the women I really like would give me a second glance." Michael hid from this painful belief, and his expectation of rejection, with mild drunkenness, absorbing computer games and a lot of food.

MELANIE

Melanie was also unsettled by her list of beliefs. It made her even more aware of the uneven balance of work at home, especially when she had to look after her mother as well. She wanted to blame her husband for not helping out more, but she was the one putting everyone else's needs before her own. It put her at the centre of family life. She was needed.

When Melanie considered what life would be like without her reward feasts she immediately experienced a sense of injustice. She had already given up so much of herself that it just seemed unfair that she should have to give this up too. Without these rewards, Melanie felt she would be completely overwhelmed by the demands of her family. But she had to concede that her kids were old enough now to do more for themselves, and that she was perfectly capable of negotiating a better arrangement with her husband.

Melanie's dread was the possibility that she might not really be needed at all. Her central belief was: "If I stop doing everything for my family, I will become invisible." It frightened her.

KATIE

Katie faced her own quandary. She adores her family. They are her best friends. She would do anything to avoid hurting them, so she was already aware of her dread as she imagined changing her lifestyle. She even wondered about getting a place of her own but knew she would miss them all too much.

Katie saw how her friends lived, and she liked the healthy food they ate when she visited them. She envied how fit they were, not just their slimness. She wanted to try some changes, but felt her family's lifestyle was an insurmountable obstacle. Her dread beliefs were: "I believe my parents would feel hurt if I refused their food and decided to do my own thing. I believe they would feel I was rejecting everything they have done for me throughout my life." Katie knew she would never do anything that would hurt her family's feelings.

Perhaps you identify with Michael, Melanie or Katie, perhaps not. You will have your own unique story, your own unique beliefs and your own unique fear of change. You need to be aware of what it is you are dealing with before you can change. Understanding a problem properly is usually more than half the battle; this is the hard work of real change. Once you know your own picture, and all its complicating factors, it is time to look at the picture you really want.

IMAGINE A DIFFERENT PICTURE

It is well known that the future someone visualises in their mind, good or bad, is more likely to come to pass than one that is not foreseen at all (earthquakes and lightening strikes notwithstanding). There is nothing mystical about this. The mind has simply created a destination, and will start to spot opportunities from the surrounding world to help take you there. This mechanism only works, however, when the destination is reachable. Self-help books often try to emulate this by asking readers to write out all their hopes and dreams for the future as freely as possible. The pitfall of this approach is that many people come up with a kind of utopia: a winning-the-lottery sort of future that bears no relation to their actual lives. On the other hand, there is little point in visualising a future that is unduly modest in its ambitions. A better option is the middle way; one that is neither too extravagant nor too timid about the possibilities.

Imagine a future where you have resolved just two things: whatever it is that you dread when you think about the changes needed to help you lose weight for good; and being overweight itself. Everything else stays the same. You will not be transported to some uber-glamorous life, nor will you suddenly become fabulously wealthy. You will still have to go to work, there will still be ironing to do, winters will still be cold and wet. But in this ordinary vision of an alternative life, you have conquered your dread and you are a healthy weight.

It is not as simple as it sounds. If all you have ever fantasised about is how low a number you can reach on the scales, or getting into all those smaller clothes you have packed away, then this will be a much bigger vision to pull together. You may struggle to bring it in to focus but persevere. It will mean imagining things that might seem impossible at present, but do not worry about the real world for now. In your own mind you have the freedom to reconstruct the future you want.

If it helps, imagine a version of yourself living in a parallel universe. To all intents and purposes, he or she lives exactly the same life that you do. It is not perfect; he or she may still be strapped for cash, or worry about how the kids are doing at school, but they are free of the dread-belief that trips you up in your world, and they are a healthy weight. What does this life look like? How does it go on a day-to-day basis? How are key relationships changed? What new skills, new places and new faces emerge in this vision that are not in your real life?

MICHAEL

When Michael thought about a perfect future he put himself on a yacht cruising the Greek islands with a beautiful wife and a couple of cute children. In this vision, he had the physique of Superman, great wealth, a huge high-tech house and plenty of leisure time. It is fun to daydream like this from time to time, but there is such a gulf between this and real life that the mind cannot grasp it as anything other than a fantasy. Michael's perfect future is so unreal it cannot not ruffle the feathers of his subconscious. So buckling down to the task in hand, Michael came up with a more real, yet strangely more intimidating vision of the future. In this future he only addressed two things: the absence of a loving partner and being overweight.

He imagined a leaner version of himself going to work, but coming home to a lovely partner instead of his computer screen. He saw a life that was full of possibilities within this new and special companionship. He added in all the things he really wanted: intimate evenings at home, going to concerts, going on holiday with his partner, having friends over. The evenings of computer games, beer and fast-food were swept aside.

He realised he would go home from work earlier if this were the case, and that he sometimes created additional work for himself in order to avoid going home. But he also saw that he got his senior position because he was good at his job, not because his physical bulk made an impression.

Michael imagined himself as a fit man who played football with his friends and held his own as a member of their team. In his mind, he also turned himself a runner. He often looked at the lean men who ran past him in the street in all their gear and smart trainers and wondered how it was possible to be like that.

Michael smiled as he thought of this fine picture, but he felt the old anxiety rising. He heard the familiar and cruel belief: "No decent girl will ever want a big fat guy like me. I am out of my depth with this." Nevertheless, he was aware that some sort of genie had been let out of a bottle – this alternative vision of the future, where he still lived his own life but with just these two changes. And every time the old beliefs reared their heads, he thought about this different life.

MELANIE

Melanie found it very hard to see a different future of any kind, even a fantasy version. She always tried to accept the things she could not change, and it certainly felt like this applied to her present life. The thing she wanted more than anything was the one thing she knew she could never have; she wished she could go back to a time when her kids were little and loved and needed her so much. This is Melanie's fantasy future, the equivalent of Michael's yacht. But at least she recognised that part of her 'wrong' picture was that she was struggling to come to terms with her children growing up. They would be leaving home soon, and Melanie was not sure who she would be then. Her own life had been on hold for so long that she had lost sight of it.

Melanie started to wonder what it might be like if the family loved and needed her without all this hard work. What if they appreciated her even if she just sat on the sofa all day? She cautiously put together a vision of the future where the family pitched in with the housework, and the kids went along to help their grandmother sometimes. In this future, they all remembered birthdays and anniversaries without any prompting, and her children sought her company for its own sake. Melanie also saw this was a future where they took more responsibility as they made the transition to adult life, and where she helped them with that, instead of babying them.

She still could not imagine a slim version of herself in this future. Apart from anything else, what would she do with all that free time? She would probably eat even more. As she thought about it, though, other possibilities started to fill the time. She could see her own friends again; she could take her mother somewhere nice instead of just resentfully cleaning her house; she and her husband could do more together; and she could get back to gardening. Instead of just sitting and eating all day, Melanie realised she would have time to attend to her health.

As Melanie thought about this future, the dread came back to her. If she stopped doing everything, would they all just ignore her? It felt like a kind of death.

KATIE

In Katie's fantasy future, she looked like a model with long legs and a huge wardrobe full of designer clothes and shoes. It was the only vision she had ever held and she knew it wasn't real. What would she actually look like 60 lbs lighter? She could not see a slim version of herself watching television as her family tucked into snacks while she did not. It seemed like she had to choose between her health and her family.

Katie decided to fast-forward a bit to a time where she and a partner were raising a family in a home of their own. She saw an image where she was in charge of family meals. Katie wanted to protect her future children from the bullying she and her brothers had faced at school because they were overweight. She wanted them to be fit and healthy so they could run about and play with the other children, and not be excluded as she had been.

As Katie created this vision in her head, she realised she was replicating the home of one of her friends. Sharon also comes from a close family but they are all slim. Katie has eaten with them many times, and their meals are very different from those at her house. They are smaller but better and healthier, and there is no snacking in front of the television. In fact Sharon's family don't really sit in front of the television at all; they are all off doing other things. Katie wanted this for her own family in the future.

As she saw this future in her head, Katie realised how little control she had over what she ate at home. When she tried to imagine taking more control by refusing some of her parent's meals, or making her own, she could see the hurt look on their faces. It upset her. Yet she could not dislodge this new image of raising her own family, and being in charge of their health and her own.

This may seem like just a bit of daydreaming, but it is not. If you have judged this correctly, along the middle way, you should have a vision of something that is genuinely achievable, even if you cannot quite see how you might achieve it at this point. This is your destination. You have just created the most important and powerful tool to break the dread-belief that is holding you back. This altered version of the future is one that your conscious mind is fully in charge of, whether your subconscious likes it or not. Every time the dread appears, present it with your new vision of the future. Your subconscious will be saying: "Don't kid yourself, this is impossible." Your conscious mind must reply: "But this is what I really want." And now you are about to up the ante.

ADDING PRESSURE TO BREAK WRONG BELIEFS

I hope by now you can see how your existing beliefs are influencing your behaviour, and producing outcomes in your life that you may not want. If you have worked through the steps above, you will already have opened up your mind to new possibilities. You have started to set the scene for you own triggering event.

At this point, you may feel that, while your beliefs have had a good shaking under all this scrutiny, and have been dented with a fresh picture of the future, they have by no means gone away. Indeed, your subconscious will almost certainly be protecting your existing beliefs with a long list of 'ifs' and 'buts', and telling you that change is too difficult. Do not to try to work out how your new future might come about just yet. Do not give your subconscious anything to get hold of. Just answer its tug with your new vision of the future.

Self-help aficionados might think this is another version of 'positive thinking' but it is not. I am not a big fan of positive thinking, it is often just an avoidance tactic. I am a much stronger advocate of facing reality, warts and all; in this case, seeing the negative impact of obstructing beliefs about your health and being overweight. The point of creating a vision of a better future is not to whitewash difficult beliefs, it is to directly challenge them. You need to notice when these old beliefs are firing, so that you can confront them, not suppress them with 'positive' blinkers.

The next step is to give your conscious mind an extra boost with a set of tools that will help you apply constant pressure on the subconscious.

What if you are wrong?

This harks back to my earlier comments regarding the importance of recasting apparent 'truths' as beliefs. You can change beliefs but you probably will not even try to change something you perceive as a truth, because you will not think it possible.

It is a difficult transition to make, especially where a big hitter 'truth' has governed your life for a long time. This switch from: "It is true that.." to "I only believe that.." can take time and patience. Once you admit that the obstacles you face are only beliefs, the obvious question is: "What if I am wrong?" Accepting this possibility will greatly undermine a belief by introducing doubt. Doubt is an essential, early ingredient of belief-breaking.

If you have held something to be true for a long time, it may be rather embarrassing to admit that you might have been wrong all along. If you have stuck to a position defiantly, or dismissively, in the past, it may seem like you could lose face if you change your position now. Consider the consequences, though, of staying loyal to a belief that you are no longer sure of, for the sake of your pride. It keeps you trapped in a place where you no longer want to be.

It is difficult to wonder if your beliefs are wrong without pondering the alternatives. What might be the case instead? If your answer to that question is not clear, or even non-existent, then your next task is to fill in the blank. This opens the mind up to the real possibility of doing things differently.

Gathering evidence against your beliefs

Gathering evidence against the belief, or beliefs, that you want to dispel is much more than asking yourself if they might be wrong. It is moving on to the work of convincing yourself of this. Remember that it is just two things that you altered in your new vision of the future: the thing you dreaded most if you changed the behaviours that contribute to your being overweight; and being overweight itself. You must remain focused on these two things for this exercise.

You need to think of everything you can that rationally opposes the beliefs that are keeping you tied to a way of life that no longer works for you. You may be surprised by how easy it is to do this. For example, if you continue to believe that it is impossible to lose a lot of weight and keep it off, then the existence of 10,000 members of the National Weight Control Registry, who all managed to do this, proves you wrong. If they can do it, why can't you? Moreover, the number of people who remain slim but live perfectly content lives without overeating shows it is possible to be happy without excess food.

If you believe that someone who is overweight will struggle to find a partner, then note how many people are overweight but happily married, and who got married while they were overweight. If you believe that only slim people get promotion, look at how many overweight managers there are at your workplace or who hold public office. If you believe that the only way to handle the stress in your life is to compensate with overeating, then consider those whose lives are just as stressful but handle this differently and remain slim.

These counter-arguments need to be quite calculating. It is a bit like cross-examining yourself in a court of law. What evidence is admissible or inadmissible? Emotionally berating yourself is absolutely inadmissible, because this would be gathering evidence against yourself, not evidence against your beliefs. Your inability to stop overeating on the grounds that you just like food too much does not count. It is not relevant, because everyone likes food. One correct counter-argument states that there is a huge range of truly wonderful food that can be eaten while regaining health. Another states that most slim people follow a taste-over-volume rule of thumb, that allows them to fully enjoy food without overeating.

In the previous chapter, I provided some counter-arguments for other common beliefs that link food with love or celebration, or questioned typical beliefs about waste or gender. Use as much evidence against your beliefs as you can come up with. You can be pretty creative with this. Basically, you are telling your subconscious that these old beliefs it clings to make no sense, over and over again.

Reverse psychology - extreme versions of old beliefs

Another way of highlighting an illogical belief is to consider an extreme version of it. For example, if you tend to respond to stress with episodes of overeating because you believe that excess food can relieve stress, then respond with an overt version of this: "All my problems in life will be solved if I just eat enough pizza." Clearly this is nonsense, yet it is consistent with the core belief you are trying to eradicate.

Anxiety about finding a partner, generates the extreme position of: "No one would ever accept me as a partner because I have absolutely no other qualities apart from being overweight." Anyone reading that statement must surely see at once how absurd it is. This should bring the additional benefit of making you realise just how many good qualities you do have, and how much you have to offer a partner.

Those who believe that they simply do not have the energy to increase their physical activity, might want to try something like: "I will be completely traumatised if I even try to walk round the garden." Once you get the hang of this, it can be quite good fun. You are pulling you own leg, but your subconscious will still be listening.

Finding the antidote belief

Sometimes identifying the opposite position of a belief can expose its weakness. These antidote beliefs are not always that easy to find but they can be powerful. Care is needed, however, to avoid creating greater absurdity or confusion.

If you believe that love, nurturing and food are deeply entwined – that food is about loving - the opposite may seem to be that food is about hating. This doesn't work. It does not expose the absurdity of the food-love belief. It just introduces another absurd belief. Food is *not* love is the correct opposite here, and it gains traction as "food is *never* love", because love is love. This statement is absolutely true and hopefully your common sense will see it at once. You need to find the opposite that works therefore, not one that is equally illogical.

Perhaps you hold a belief that healthy food is boring. The two possible opposites are: "Healthy food is not boring," or, "Healthy food is wonderful." These are fine but not that compelling. The original belief may have its roots in many years of dull dieting food. This should not be confused with what I can only call 'real' food, with which many repeat dieters are unfamiliar. The troublesome belief is actually: "diet food is boring," and so it is. Its antidote belief is better expressed as: "real food is wonderful," where this is distinguished from diet food, as well as high-calorie baked foods and ultra-processed convenience food.

It is probably worth looking at: "Fast-food tastes wonderful," using the term to include all ultra-processed meals and snacks. As I mentioned in an earlier chapter, fast-food is formulated to be highly palatable and habit-forming. If someone only eats fast-food or dull diet food, they may have little experience of the much better food that sits between these two extremes. This may make it difficult to spot the correct antidote belief, which is: "fast-food is monotonous." It is greasy, clawing, over salted or excessively sweet. Real food, on the other hand, offers a wide range of flavours and sensual experiences. It is also wonderfully nutritious. There is really no contest here.

Some opposite beliefs bring their own insights. A belief that states: "Potential partners will reject me because I am fat," could become: "Potential partners will not reject me because I am fat." There is some purchase in that, because plenty of potential partners would not. A different opposite, however, is: "Potential partners may reject me when I am slim." This is thornier because, of course, it is true. Being slim brings no guarantee of potential partners queuing up to be with you. It forces you to think about who you really are, and what it is you have to offer a partner, whether you are overweight or not.

This prospect will lift the spirits of some but not all. If you have spent many years believing that being overweight is the reason you do not have a partner, then imagining a scenario where a slim version of yourself could still be rejected is unsettling. You would not be able to blame being overweight anymore. You may feel oddly vulnerable without your excess weight, and this might not be something you have ever considered before. But slim people face their share of unrequited love. This is just life.

The point of this approach is to search for an opposing version of a belief until you find the one that is exposing its absurdity. These tactics may seem like trivial mind games but they unmask tenuous beliefs nonetheless. Used cleverly, they can create the additional pressure needed to put a wrong belief under stress, and force your common sense to see it for what it is.

The contrast between present life and new vision

Once something is seen it cannot be unseen. You will find it difficult to ignore the new possibilities that you have created in your mind. Every time you do something 'old style', such as overeating, you will notice, even if you are not quite ready to stop yet. You might annoy yourself with this, but it is all grist to the mill. You may say to yourself: "I don't want this anymore," or "I want to be free of this," or, importantly "I deserve a better life than this." Your subconscious will be listening.

Creating 'gain' beliefs

In an earlier chapter, I noted that those who succeeded in losing weight, and maintaining this over long periods, held beliefs that were framed in terms of what they stood to gain, not what they were losing. This shift of emphasis matters a great deal. It is much easier to keep travelling towards a positive goal than to wearily soldier on carrying a sense of deprivation on your shoulders. Moreover, the subconscious responds more to achieving messages than sacrificing ones.

You should be able to define 'gain' beliefs that are customised to your own circumstances. Instead of seeing a future deprived of all your favourite foods, or just far too much food generally, see a future in which you are free from anxiety about being overweight. This enables you to replace a belief that says: "I will never be able to eat like this again," with something like "I am breaking free from this unhappiness." Other gain beliefs include:

- I am reclaiming my health

- I am in charge of the food, the food is not in charge of me

- I am treating my body with tenderness and respect

- I am becoming the best version of myself

- I am returning home to my true self

Sometimes much deeper issues emerge. This can include a hidden ambivalence about life itself. Many people who openly abuse their health, for example with alcohol or drugs, do not care that much if they live or die. They are not suicidal in any ordinary sense, they are just not that bothered about their future. This justifies the self-abuse. There are other subtler versions of this, such as smoking cigarettes, a habit of reckless driving or, for some, overeating to the point of obesity. This is a sobering issue but it is obviously important. It forces someone to ask themselves how much they really want to live and, if they do, how well they want to live. It is the source of the most powerful gain belief of all:

I am saving my own life.

The gain beliefs you choose must feel right for you, they must strike a real chord within you, if they are to be effective. This distinguishes them from the lists of affirmations so beloved by 'positive thinkers', who tend to use statements like this to plaster over difficult truths. The switch in perspective from loss to gain is sincere, it is not a pretence or an avoidance tactic. You must face up to the difficulties in your life if you are to successfully address them.

'Act as if'

Basically, this approach means 'acting as if' you are already living within the altered vision of your future. It sounds deceptively simple. I have left it to the end because it needs courage. Sometimes you have to prove to your subconscious that the terrible outcome it believes is the inevitable consequence of a new behaviour is neither inevitable nor terrible. It means putting your dread-belief to a direct test. This is extremely powerful but not for the faint hearted. It is the theory behind treatments for phobias, sometimes called 'flood therapy'. The idea is to expose someone to the thing they are most terrified of, bit by bit, until they calm down. 'Act as if' is not as extreme as exposure to a phobia, but it does mean directly confronting your fears.

If someone overeats to compensate for a sparse social life, 'act as if' would mean taking the brave step of getting out there to meet new people and expand their social horizons. Someone who dreads the physical exposure of visiting a public swimming pool would just go anyway. They would, no doubt, discover that no one notices them, and that lots of other overweight people are there too. If someone feels stressed by patronising co-workers, 'act as if' would mean confronting this directly, and asking them to show more respect. Or it could mean forcing yourself to throw all surplus food in the rubbish bin instead of eating it, even if this feels horribly wasteful. It would make you see the solution is to stop buying so much in the first place.

In the context of someone who treats themselves to a lot of fast-food as an act of self-compassion, this approach would see them forego this to see what happens. It would mean noticing what fills the space normally occupied by the food. Boredom? Anger? Self-pity? What belief lies behind these feelings?

MICHAEL

Michael, you will recall, is 36 and a senior manager at an IT firm. He has been overweight most of his adult life and lives alone. He spends his free time playing computer games and eating a lot of fast-food washed down with beer. His Saturdays are spent in the pub watching TV football with a couple of friends. He wants to settle down and raise a family but dreads facing rejection from women, perhaps even their ridicule, because he is so overweight.

Michael imagined a future where he was fit and healthy and had a lovely wife, even though this still seemed implausible. The endless evenings in front of his computer were getting to him, but he had to admit that thinking about all this had pulled his head out of the sand. He realised nothing would change until he did.

As Michael thought about his assumption that he would be automatically rejected by women because he was overweight, he allowed himself to consider the possibility that he could be wrong. What if he had already missed getting to know some great women because he was always hiding at home playing computer games? Because the more he did this, night after night, the more annoyed he was becoming with himself.

He considered what evidence he really had to support his assumption that he would be rejected? He had always been popular after all, and always made friends easily. He got on well with his colleagues, and he got promotion largely because of his social skills. People sought his advice because he was generous and supportive. He had also had girlfriends before, though admittedly they had been friends for a long time first.

Michael saw that being overweight had started to consume his whole life, not just his body. His entire lifestyle was being dictated to him because of this. He was presenting himself to the world as: "I am a fat man and nothing but a fat man," rather than "I am a great guy with a lot to offer." Michael defined himself as an overweight man and this shocked him. When he wondered if he was really that unlovable, it hit home how hard he was being on himself. He thought: "I am a loving guy, and I could be a good partner or husband, given the chance."

Self-conscious about his size, Michael knew that he could be defensive with women and wondered what would happen if he changed. He was not brave enough to go beyond this, but he was curious about what impact it would have if he just let his natural friendliness come across for a change.

MELANIE

Melanie, who is 48, works in a supermarket and lives with her husband and two teenagers. She has also been thinking about her future. Every time she ran from one chore to the next, she wondered what would happen if she just stopped. The three of them would have to shop, cook, keep the place clean and get themselves from A to B without her. Would they really stop loving her just because they had to do this?

Melanie thought back to a time when she would not have coped without some help. When she had two young babies, a

114

part-time job, and a husband working away from home, she would not have survived without her mother's support. Then there was the year her husband had been made redundant. She had to work full time, and he ran the house. He did things his own way but it was fine: the kids were happy, clean, fed and got their homework done. Nobody loved her less because she wasn't running after them, so why should they now?

Melanie had been worried that she might become invisible unless she kept doing everything for her family, but she wondered if she might actually become more visible if she stopped. It would certainly get their attention. The more Melanie thought about this, the more she wanted the new life she had imagined. And she wanted to be well enough to enjoy it, not almost disabled with breathlessness because she was so unfit.

As Melanie considered what would happen if she stopped running after the family, she realised this had already crept into her behaviour. She had not tidied the kids' rooms that week, and when she went to her mother's house she just sat and talked to her. It made her mother really happy.

KATIE

Katie, who is 24 and lives with her parents and two younger brothers, has become aware of how little control she has over what she eats. No one is holding her down and forcing food into her mouth, yet there is an element of emotional blackmail around food within the family.

As Katie looked round their living room, while they all tucked into yet another enormous meal, she realised she did not want this for herself anymore. Her friends and their families managed to live differently, so why couldn't she? She saw that being part of a happy, loving family did not depend on the amount of food being served or consumed.

Katie pictured the family in ten years time, all still living at home, and all of them three times their current size. She found this image both comical and disturbing, but the idea that her family would disown her if she changed what she ate seemed absurd. Might the family actually support her? She was doubtful.

When Katie imagined her own home, and her own healthy family, it seemed like the free side of a cage. Yet, Katie could only predict sulks and arguments with her family if she tried to make changes. Her mother, in particular, would resist this, though Katie had made subtle changes already: she noticed what her slim co-workers ate at lunchtime, and she was paying more attention to the food served at her friends' houses; she sometimes left food on her plate, and she was taking it easy with the snacks. Her family had not noticed. Katie was going under the radar.

THE MIND READY FOR A TRIGGERING EVENT

Michael, Melanie and Katie went about their lives as before. Few noticed the modest changes they had made. They had all taken time to define their beliefs, and saw how they influenced day to day life. Each of them had also reached a point where they knew they wanted to change.

This process can take a few weeks of conscious effort, sometimes longer. Do not be disheartened if there is no miraculous change within a few days. Your old beliefs will try to hang on, so this final stage may need a bit of patience and persistence. If you have come this far, you will have started to prepare your mind for change. You may feel you are almost there, especially if you have a good grasp of what it is you most dread, but also of its absurdity. With a new vision of the future, you have already started to change direction, and this puts more pressure on old beliefs.

By sustaining this pressure, your mind will automatically scan for more evidence to challenge the status quo. Your attention will be drawn to relevant points in magazines, films, social media, passing conversations, etc, which cumulatively will start to build a lot of pressure. In this frame of mind, you will be primed for you own triggering event. It may be something dramatic, but probably it will not be. It is like a bubble that needs just one more thing to make it burst, in order to dispel old beliefs for good.

Usually this happens in a single moment, but occasionally triggering events unfold over several days; they are no less powerful for it. It may even be two different events occurring at roughly the same time that, combined, will shed new light on the issue in question. There are no rules about what form a triggering event takes, but the impact is unmistakable. A breakthrough event like this brings a surge of recognition and clarity about what needs to be done. You will feel its strength. A true triggering event will set you free, and there is no going back.

You will find your own 'hook' within this moment. A hook reaches out to you from the future and pulls you towards your new destination. It might be a phrase or an image, or a combination of both, like a motto only stronger. A guiding light, your hook will represent your determination to live differently from now on. It may be quite meaningless to others, but your hook will speak right to your heart.

Triggering events can be very private. It may be difficult to explain to others that you have experienced a big shift in your thinking, especially in the early days. Those close to you may be unsettled by the changes you make; they may even be dismissive. You may want to give yourself time to get used to your new mindset before discussing it with others.

On the other hand, there are some people who will want to tell everyone about this big change in their lives. It is understandable and it is a personal decision. Whichever camp you fall into, do not try to talk someone round to your new way of thinking. "Beware the zeal of the new convert," as the old saying goes. Enthusiasm is wonderful, but health evangelism can be annoying. Share your optimism with others when you are ready, but avoid forcing it onto them.

Do not be tempted to feign a triggering event, or try to convince yourself that some passing event counts as a trigger. You will not have to persuade yourself of the significance of a true triggering event; it will be perfectly clear. Crucially, they are moments of positive resolve, and never moments of angry resolve in response to despair or self-loathing.

Recall Robert Fritz' elastic string model from the previous chapter, that sprung someone back from escalating weight gain onto a crash diet in a moment of panic.[62] These are not triggering events, they are just moments of panic that gloss over obstructing beliefs. For example, a forthcoming family event may be the spur for an episode of weight-loss, and may seem to be some sort of triggering event. In fact, this is just a manifestation of: "I believe my body is something to be ashamed of." This particular belief has a lurking twin: "If I do not sustain a sense of shame about my body, I will lose the motivation to lose weight." They are nasty little beliefs, and both should be discarded.

Beliefs that generate self-loathing are never right. They will always produce wrong outcomes. You no more need a sense of shame to reclaim your health than you need your house to go on fire. Your body needs your compassion and tenderness, not your hatred or anger.

Beware the tripwire here. Do not hoodwink yourself into believing that this kind of tenderness includes baking yourself a tray of cupcakes, or buying treat food because you have had a tough day. This is a food-treats-stress position. You need to cleave the two apart. Face up to the stress but keep on track with your journey home to health; both are acts of compassion towards yourself.

MICHAEL

Michael thought about his situation over a few weeks. He now understood what had been holding him back from the future he wanted, but he felt frustrated that he had not worked out how to make bigger changes. He still came home to his empty apartment, switched on his computer, put a ready-meal in the microwave and opened a beer.

Then one evening, after getting in from work, he went to turn on his computer as usual, but stopped. He looked at the machine waiting for him to waste another evening of his life, and he just turned around and walked straight back out the front door. He had no idea where he was going; he just started walking. He decided he would keep walking, rather than go back and sit at the computer. And as he walked, he though about the future he wanted so much.

Michael broke out of his reverie when he realised it was getting dark. He checked his watch and realised that he had been walking for over two hours. He had not thought he was capable of this; he was not even out of breath. He was astonished. "I can do this," he thought. He suddenly realised that all he had to do to reach a different future was to keep walking towards it. This became Michael's hook. As he headed home, he knew this was his turning point; he would walk in the evenings instead of sitting at his computer. This simple solution made everything possible. He would regain his health and reduce his weight. Maybe, in a while, he could start some running. He would regain his self-confidence, and that, of course, would change everything.

MELANIE

Melanie became increasingly wistful about all the things she would do if she had the time. She worried there would be arguments if she just stopped doing everything, however, so she carried on. The evenings of feasting continued, though she looked at all this unnecessary food and wondered if she would ever stop overeating. She tried to stick to small snacks, but could not resist going back and forth to the fridge for more food. It seemed nothing much had changed at all.

Then her car broke down. The repair was going to cost more than the car was worth so Melanie decided to scrap it, even though she could not afford a new one. A family conference followed. Melanie could get a lift to work, but her son and daughter would have to fend for themselves and sort out their social lives. No more mummy-chauffeur. And they just accepted it. Melanie had not expected the loss of her car to free up so much of her time, but it did.

A few days later, an old gardening friend came into the supermarket where she worked and invited Melanie to her allotment for tea. Melanie felt a wave of nostalgia when she saw all the gardeners tending their plants, but hesitated when her friend told her that one of the plots had become free. It needed a lot of work, and Melanie knew she was not fit enough to take it on. When she told the family that evening, however, her husband and son immediately volunteered to do the heavy work to get things started, and her daughter offered to spruce up the little shed, and help with the planting.

The following weekend Melanie was standing in her own allotment watching her family help her get this project off the ground. Just two weeks earlier she would not have thought this possible. As she cleared away some dead wood, she noticed one piece that had some new shoots, and she realised it was time for her to come back to life too. Suddenly, Melanie saw that she was standing in the first scene of her new future, and knew that she would never go back to the old way of doing things.

KATIE

Katie was also starting to think that there was no way out of her predicament. The small changes she had made seemed like a drop in the ocean. When she discovered she has gone up another dress size, however, she plucked up the courage to weight herself. She had gained another 25 lbs in six months; she was 227 lbs. This time she did not slide into panic, or phone her mum for reassurance. She just looked in the mirror and asked herself: "If this is what I am like now, what will I be like in ten years time?" This question became Katie's hook. In that moment, she saw that she needed to save her own life.

Katie knew at once this did not just mean lengthening her life; it meant reaching out for the life she had pictured in her head for the past few weeks. That was the life she was saving. Katie finally realised she might have to choose between that life and her family. With all her heart, she hoped they would support her but, if they did not, she would still choose life. And she realised that this was the first truly adult decision she had ever made.

You will have your own story, and your own hook, to pull you towards a better future. It is the thing that will keep you on track, or get you back on track after a slip, and there will be occasional slips. The old temptations will lure you from time to time. You will feel their tug, but your new mindset will intervene. Your own personal hook will help you dust yourself off and carry on, instead of giving up in despair.

A FUNDAMENTAL LIFE DECISION

In his book, *The Path of Least Resistance*, Robert Fritz makes the distinction between fundamental life decisions and primary or secondary decisions. He argues that primary decisions relate to discrete projects in our lives, even if they are quite long-term. This includes nurturing a career, establishing a lovely home, learning to be a good cook or travelling round the world. Secondary decisions support primary ones: applying for promotion, choosing the décor for your home or ingredients for a special meal, and so on. In day-to-day life, we mostly focus on our primary and secondary decisions.

Fundamental decisions, or fundamental commitments, function at a higher level; they have greater overarching meaning in our lives. For example, someone may make the fundamental decision to live to their highest potential; a primary decision may follow that involves selecting a career path consistent with their best qualities and strengths. An artist may make the fundamental commitment to being the central creative force in his or her life, and translate this into various creative projects. A doctor may fulfil a fundamental commitment to serve his or her community by trying to restore the health of others.

It is possible to make primary choices in life without the back-up of a fundamental life decision. For example, someone may attend a place of worship, and follow certain religious rituals, without ever making a fundamental decision to embrace and serve God. Someone may get married and have children, without making a fundamental decision to live within a committed relationship. Such discrepancies may also be found around political or financial decisions and, of course, decisions about health. Such commitments are weakened, however, if they are not based on fundamental decisions.

Health needs a fundamental decision. It is not enough to decide to join a gym, or eat more fresh vegetables, or try the latest diet. At best, these are weak primary and secondary decisions. A fundamental decision about your health means a full commitment to your physical and mental heath for life. It is the decision to do everything you can to experience the joy of being as well as possible, for as long as possible. Because what is the alternative?

Epilogue

This process placed Michael, Melanie and Katie at the start of a life-long journey to better health. They all took their new paths towards different, better lives and joined the ranks of the long-term, weight-loss maintainers.

There are no guarantees in life, but creating the life you truly want is only possible in the presence of supportive beliefs, and with a clear vision of where you want to go. The essential changes needed for your health and happiness, then, need no longer be hostage to anxious hope, but part of a committed decision about how things will be from now on.

I could have ended on that note, but something made me hesitate. The human body has what, in evolutionary terms, is a safety net. In the modern era of obesity, however, it has become a tripwire. If you are unaware of it then you may well trip over it, and that would be a great shame, especially if it injured your faith in newly formed beliefs. I mentioned earlier that I strongly advocate gradual weight loss, and now I want to explain why this is so important. Although the central point of this book is the powerful role our beliefs play in our lives, it is still prudent to have a good knowledge of how the body responds to weight loss that is too rapid. Forewarned is forearmed. So let me tell you a story....

THE MINNESOTA SEMI-STARVATION EXPERIMENT, 1944

Towards the end of the Second World War, Professor Ancel Keys, and his colleagues at Minnesota University, recruited 36 healthy, male conscientious objectors to participate in a study of human starvation.[63] In 1944, the Allied Forces were entering what had been German-occupied cities across Europe, and, in some, found emaciated civilian populations living on little more than potatoes and scraps of bread.

At the time, there was little scientific knowledge about human starvation, or how to safely and rapidly re-feed people who had suffered such extreme deprivation. The American War Department asked Keys and his team to assess the physical and psychological impact of starvation, and to identify the most efficient method of rehabilitation. A brief study of starvation had been conducted towards the end of the First World War but it had only studied 12 volunteers. This was useful, but it was considered too small a study to give the conclusive answers needed to tackle the widespread hunger across Europe in 1944.[64]

The 36 volunteers escaped the draft on the grounds of their conscientious objection to killing others, but they willingly committed to this gruelling experiment, aware that their countrymen were risking their lives trying to liberate Europe. They would need their strong resolve. For the 12-month study, they lived together in an open dormitory under the close supervision of the research team, and were subjected to many physical and psychological tests.

The men were all aged 25-33 and were neither overweight nor underweight at the start of the study. For the first 12 weeks, they all received a maintenance diet of around 3000 kcals per day, so that baseline observations could be taken. During the following 24 weeks this ration was halved to 1500 kcals per day (the equivalent of 1000 kcals per day for women). In addition, the men had to walk for at least 22 miles per week. The researchers adjusted each man's rations to ensure they all lost roughly 2.5 lbs every week. At the end of this period, all of the men had lost around a third of their body weight (around 50-60 lbs).

The impact of this rapid weight loss on these previously healthy young men was meticulously documented. General weakness, and a reduction in muscular strength, were unsurprising, early effects. As time passed, the daily walks became more and more exhausting, and previously simple tasks, such as opening heavy doors, became difficult. The men also reported feeling cold all the time and requested extra blankets at night, even at the height of summer. Despite their carefully controlled diets, they became anaemic and their metabolisms slowed down; their total energy expenditure fell by half during this period of the study. They reported extreme fatigue, lethargy, dizziness and reduced co-ordination, and there was a marked loss of sex drive. The researchers also noted that shaving wounds healed more slowly, nails grew slowly, and the men's hair started to fall out. And, of course, they were constantly hungry.

These findings were similar to those made by Francis Benedict, who conducted the First World War study in 1917. His subjects had "a constant gnawing sensation in the stomach. They found it almost impossible to keep warm, even with an excessive amount of clothing...[There was] a decrease in sexual interest and expression which, in some, reached the point of obliteration". Benedict also noted that his subjects had a 30% drop in metabolism. A kind of inertia became evident; the men were listless, and reluctant to do anything that required much physical effort, as they found it so exhausting. They reduced their activity so much that, if they consumed more than 2100 kcals a day (almost a third less than they had eaten previously), they would begin to regain weight.

It was the psychological impact on these mentally robust young men, however, that Ancel Keys found particularly striking, even though they had been hand-picked to cope with the rigors of the experiment. They became increasingly irritable with and intolerant of one another. One participant later recalled that he was shocked at the strength of hatred he felt towards those who were free to eat normally.[65] Some had to withdraw from the university courses that they had signed up for because they simply did not have the motivation or concentration to continue. A visiting journalist noted the men had lost all drive and ambition. Their interests had narrowed and few things could stir them to action – all characteristics of premature ageing.

All of the men became obsessed with food. They began to daydream about food, and it became a constant topic of conversation. Some began collecting recipe books, and poured over them compulsively. Others developed rituals in order to eek out their food rations: they diluted the food, or sucked tiny pieces of it to make it last longer. Initially, the men had been allowed chewing gum but this was withdrawn when it was noted that some were getting through up to 40 packets a day. One recalled the frustration of constantly thinking about food:

> "It made food the most important thing in one's life…..It became the one central and only thing in one's life. And life is pretty dull if that's the only thing. I mean, if you went to a movie, you weren't particularly interested in the love scenes, but you noticed every time they ate and what they ate."

One subject broke down after eight weeks, and binged on ice-cream, milk shakes and candy. When challenged he started "weeping and making threats of violence". Another broke at seven weeks with "a sudden and complete loss of willpower and ate several cookies, a bag of popcorn and two bananas before he could regain control of himself". One of the greatest legacies of this experiment was the discovery that rapid weight loss directly and predictably affects the mind and personality as well as the body.

All these consequences came from losing just 2.5 lbs a week. Yet, this is exactly what many modern-day slimming diets recommend. Some of the more extreme diets aim for up to 7 lbs of weight loss per week. If the story so far is not enough to persuade you to question the credibility of these diets, then perhaps what happened next will.

At the end of the 24-week period of weight loss, the men were divided into groups to test various dietary formulas to see which one offered the most rapid restoration of energy and strength. This period of rehabilitation lasted 12 weeks, but their diets were still controlled by the research team. Various combinations of protein, fat and carbohydrate were tried, but all the diets were set at 'maintenance' levels between 2200 to 3000 kcals per day. All of the men were slow to recover. Regardless of the composition of their diet, all of them agreed they were "not back to normal" after this 3-month period. Significantly, the constant hunger persisted.

For a further 8 weeks, twelve of the men remained under observation but were allowed to eat freely. Although they were warned not to overeat, from day one they all did. One of the men ate such a large meal he had to be admitted to hospital to have his stomach pumped. Another ate several meals in one day and was sick on a bus. The men's calorie intake rose to over 8,000 a day, yet they remained perversely unsatisfied. They insisted they were still hungry, even when physically incapable of eating any more food. And they craved energy-dense food, rich in fat and carbohydrate (just like ultra-processed fast-food), which is known to produce body fat rapidly.

Weight gain was prodigious and quick (over 50 lbs in 8 weeks). By the end of this final phase, the men weighed 5% more than at the start of the experiment but had 50% more body fat. "Boy did I add weight," one of the men recalled, when interviewed some years later. "Well, that was flab. You don't have your muscle back yet." The men's recovery, by their own definitions, took from two months to two years, though none felt there were long-term negative consequences. All of them eventually returned to their pre-experiment weight and health.[66]

Benedict made similar observations in 1917. He noted: "One general feature of the post-experimental history is the excess eating immediately indulged in by the men." Despite cautions about overindulgence, the men "almost invariably overate....In particular, the cravings for sweets and snacks were now free to be indulged, and so they were". His subjects regained all their weight and body fat in less than two weeks; a week later they had gained, on average, an additional eight pounds. He wrote: "In practically every instance, the weight prior to the beginning of the experiment was reached almost immediately and was usually materially exceeded".

Nearly three decades later, Ancel Keys concluded that the composition of the diet given to someone who has endured a degree of starvation is less important than the simple provision of a lot of calories. Energy-dense food makes sense in this situation, as so many calories can be consumed in small volumes of food. His team also concluded that the semi-starved population of a war-torn country would have little drive to undertake the restorative work needed to re-establish infrastructure, until they had been adequately re-fed. As it turned out, Key's study came too late to help exhausted Europeans, but this groundbreaking study continues to be of considerable use to scientists researching obesity, weight loss, anorexia nervosa or bulimia, and the impact of famine.

Our bodies are highly adaptable. If excess weight is carried for any length of time, the body resets to accept this as 'normal'. The biological mechanisms that keep everything in balance will then protect this fatter status quo. Even if someone is significantly overweight, the body (the brain, to be precise) registers rapid weight loss as starvation and tries to correct this. It makes no difference if this is a healthy young man volunteering for a 6-month period of semi-starvation or someone who is overweight going on an excessively strict diet.

In 1997, Professor Abdul Dulloo, from the University of Geneva, revisited the data from the Minnesota experiment to see if fresh conclusions could be drawn that would be relevant to contemporary concerns about obesity.[67] Dulloo focused on the period of rehabilitation and free eating that followed semi-starvation. He identified three physiological mechanisms that kick in simultaneously when the body is working to reclaim rapidly lost weight:

- it drops the metabolic rate and restricts energy expenditure (movement)
- it replenishes lost fat before it restores muscle
- it induces powerful hunger

It is well known that the metabolic rate drops in response to rapid weight loss. Dulloo noted that it remains low until the body's fat stores have returned to pre-weight-loss levels. The drop in metabolism induces a physical inertia in order to discourage unnecessary energy expenditure. (The correct term is reduced or negative thermogenesis.) This is why people whose weight constantly goes down and up, as a result of yo-yo dieting, feel so reluctant to take exercise. It is not laziness. It is the body inducing a degree of torpor while it reclaims its fat stores.

Dulloo also noted that the men in the Minnesota experiment gained back more weight than they lost, but ended up with a much higher percentage of body fat. He concluded that the body prioritises restoration of fat and, when this has reached pre-diet levels, switches to regaining muscle mass (strictly 'fat-free mass'). But the body continues to lay down fat while it is doing this, hence the overshoot in fat and overall weight.

In order to achieve this rapid restoration of fat, the body ignites a deep and powerful hunger. The correct term for this is 'autoregulation hyperphagia' (literally excessive swallowing). Most of us would call it binge eating or compulsive eating, or even gorging. I prefer the term 'deep hunger' and anyone planning to lose weight, especially a lot of weight, needs to know about it. Deep hunger is the ultimate saboteur of long-term weight loss.

DEEP HUNGER – DO NOT WAKEN SLEEPING DOGS

The account above should bring cheer, not despair, to anyone who is overweight. Thousands of people have succeeded in maintaining significant weight loss over long periods, so the moral of the story is that it is perfectly possible to do this. My cautionary tale warns of the pitfalls of *rapid* weight loss, and its direct link to rebound weight gain. It is a sad paradox that those most desperate to lose weight can be so easily lured into the trap of rapid weight-loss diets that will then expose them to compulsive re-feeding. These diets will sentence you to a never-ending cycle of weight loss and regain that will eventually lead to obesity. The only way to break this cycle is to go under your brain's radar and lose weight gradually. It is the long game, and it works.

We have three different types of hunger. Firstly, there is appetite, which is not strictly hunger at all, but a response to the sight or anticipation of food that looks and smells pleasing. This sense will be enhanced in the presence of actual hunger, which is why lean people often delay eating in order to heighten the sensual pleasure of food.

People who have lost weight too rapidly, or who yo-yo diet, will have a heightened appetite most of the time because their bodies will be driving them to eat. This explains why many overweight people believe they "just like food too much". This is a skewed appetite response. It makes even dull food seem far more enticing than it really is. This is corrected when these weight swings are brought under control by slower but steady weight loss.

The second hunger is what I call surface hunger: it is needing breakfast in the morning, or the rumbling of an empty stomach when lunch is late. It can be mildly distracting, but it is quite easy to handle in small doses. This is why the current vogue for intermittent fasting has been so successful. The cornerstone of managing surface hunger over longer periods is eating regular, filling meals that will keep you 'not-hungry' for several hours. Meals that do this generally contain protein, a modest amount of fat, plant fibre and whole grains. The 'full' effect is enhanced if these are taken with fluid, such as soup. Experienced dieters already know this. Habits that will shoot you in the foot include: grazing eating patterns; sugared soda drinks which bypass the body's 'full' signals; diet soda drinks which cause sugar cravings; and alcohol which stimulates hunger.

The third hunger is deep hunger. This drives episodes of apparently uncontrollable overeating as the body fights to reclaim the fat it has lost, but also in response to certain types of food. Deep hunger is triggered by a complex interaction of hormones. It is beyond the scope of this book to describe how these hormones work in detail, but a brief overview may be useful.

Insulin is released by the pancreas after eating carbohydrate (sugary or starchy foods), or in anticipation of eating. Some people think insulin's only role is to reduce the glucose that is absorbed into the bloodstream from these carbohydrates. In fact, the main function of insulin is to transfer the energy from these foods into cells of the body. If the food consumed is surplus to requirements, the energy will be stored as fat in the fat cells. Insulin is a fat-making hormone.

Insulin levels rise in response to the amount of glucose absorbed, but also the speed at which it is absorbed. It will spike up sharply when a lot of 'fast' carbohydrate (refined sugar, refined flour or potato) is absorbed quickly and transformed into glucose. The sudden, spike of insulin dupes the body into thinking most of this glucose is surplus, so it dumps it into the fat cells for storage. This confused hormone response short-changes the energy needs of the rest of the body, which soon starts sending out aggrieved 'hunger' signals. This is why we often feel hungry again shortly after eating fast-food. It is why refined-carbohydrates are never that filling, and why it is possible to eat so much of them. This type of food provokes deep hunger, and this is why it seems so addictive.

Leptin is another hormone that is involved in the hunger response. It is excreted by the fat cells when adequate fat stores are detected across the body. When leptin levels rise, hunger ceases. When fat stores fall, so does leptin and hunger is induced. For reasons that are not well understood, this balancing system is disrupted in people who are very overweight. They have constantly high levels of leptin in their systems, but do not seem to experience the clear 'stop-eating' signals that lean people do. It is possible that the amount of leptin needed to shut off hunger is proportional to the amount of fat carried by the body. This would explain the higher levels found in people who are overweight. It may be that leptin levels cannot reach a 'stop-eating' level if someone's weight has passed a critical mass of fatness. Fortunately, this seems to corrects itself as weight is gradually lost. But if weight is lost too quickly, the leptin-system is likely involved in triggering autoregulation hyperphagia – the deep hunger that causes binge eating, as the body tries to reclaim its fat.

In the ordinary scheme of things, I believe that deep hunger is too strong a physical impulse to be resisted by anyone other than those with exceptional conviction. We can witness such conviction in a group of conscientious objectors who want to help thousands of starving people in Europe; we see it in those terrified by a health crisis; and we see it in those with mental health disorders such as anorexia nervosa. Nearly everyone else will crack under the strain. The smart thing, then, is to avoid putting yourself in this position in the first place.

The overview above is a considerable simplification, but it explains why gradual weight loss, and keeping insulin levels low, are so important. Generally, this means eating slow carbohydrate foods (low glycaemic-index) that are absorbed into the bloodstream gradually. This allows the energy from these foods to be used directly for the body's needs, rather than being immediately stored as fat. There are many low glycaemic-index food lists available online. Mostly, these are unrefined, wholegrain foods (oatmeal, wholemeal bread, wholegrain rice and pasta, legumes and pulses).

These ingredients are nutritious and filling. They are used to make some of the finest food in the world, such as the traditional diets of the Mediterranean, Middle East and North Africa. I think this is the best and most pleasurable way to lose weight gradually, and to discover some wonderful food along the way. Whether this approach is combined with some intermittent fasting is a matter of personal choice.

If you are new to gradual weight loss, it may take a while to get the balance right. Initial zeal may produce quicker weight loss than intended, and trigger an episode of deep hunger and compulsive eating. A ploy used by nearly all of the long-term maintainers was to have a pre-planned way of dealing with this, and other minor slips. They stayed calm and forgave themselves, but they also took immediate steps to get back on track.

If you find yourself in the grip of an all-consuming craving for energy-dense food that you are struggling to resist, then you need to out-manoeuvre it. You can do this by feeding it a decent-sized meal of protein and fat, taken with a slow-carbohydrate. You need to have this plan in place. You need to know beforehand what this meal will be so you can prepare it reasonably quickly. (A typical example might be a three-egg portion of scrambled eggs on buttered wholemeal toast, or a bowl of ham and lentil soup with buttered wholemeal toast.) The aim is to take a filling meal while keeping your insulin levels low with slow-carbohydrate food. This will give your body the energy it needs over the next few hours.

If this happens, accept that it will be a day of containing deep hunger and not a weight-reducing day. It should settle over the course of one day; you should be able to get back on track the next day. If you give in to a lot of fast carbohydrate food, such as cakes, biscuits or ultra-processed snacks and sweets, it may be difficult to prevent a sustained episode of binge eating and rapid weight regain.

Veteran dieters know all about hitting a plateau as they try to lose weight. It can cause great frustration. Some conclude that their efforts are hopeless and give up. I want to cast a very different light on the plateau, for it is actually a very encouraging sign. During plateaus, the body is resetting itself to a lower body weight, and it takes a bit of time for this to be recognised as the new 'normal'. This is exactly what you want. This is why long-term maintainers found that it became easier to keep the weight off after a year had passed, and even easier after two years. As long as you are not gaining weight during a plateau you are winning. Weight is not lost in a steady downward slope; it goes down in steps as the body gradually adapts to incrementally lower body weights. So be of good cheer, and keep going.

A weight loss of around one pound a week, averaged over a six or even twelve-month period, will put someone on track for permanent weight loss. It may be that a journey of two or even three years will be needed to reach a healthy weight. If this seems agonisingly slow, ask yourself how long it took to accumulate the excess weight in the first place. How long have you been trying and failing to correct this? Remember that even a modest drop in weight will bring considerable health benefits and a sense of wellbeing.

THREE COMMITMENTS

There are no recipes or exercise regimes in this book. I hope the principles I have outlined will be enough to help anyone create customised plans suited to their personal circumstances and budget. Most experienced dieters will have enough expertise about what does and does not work for them to be able to do this.

136

I want to end by returning to the long-term maintainers who prove so conclusively that it is possible to lose substantial amounts of weight, and live a much happier and better quality of life while sustaining this.

The typical maintainer respects his or her body with kindness and compassion. They care for their bodies with nourishing food and freedom of movement. Many reported a sense of returning home to themselves, and leaving all the despair and unhappiness behind. Our bodies are remarkably forgiving and self-healing but they need our help, so I suggest the following three commitments.

First, make the commitment that whatever weight you are now is the heaviest you will ever be, and that from this moment on your health will just get better and better.

Second, make the commitment to accept yourself just as you are right now. Give yourself the freedom to say: "This is how I am in the world today, and it is just fine." This may be difficult for someone who has hated their body for a long time, but it is important if the temptation to revert to a rapid weight-loss strategy is to be resisted.

Third, make the commitment to return home to yourself, to a place where your health has been restored and you are enjoying life, free from the burden of the dieting cycle. Every day that you nourish yourself and enjoy your body you are one step closer to home and peace. I wish you every happiness and success.

Notes and Further Reading

1 Murray C J L, et al, *Global, regional, and national prevalence of overweight and obesity in children and adults during 1980-2013: a systematic analysis for the Global Burden of Disease Study 2013*, The Lancet, May 2014.

2 Good Enough to Eat: Where in the world are the best and worst places to eat? Oxfam Report, January 2014.

3 State of the Nation's Waistline, Obesity in the UK: Analysis and Expectations, The National Obesity Forum, 2014.

4 Tackling Obesities: Future Choices – Foresight Project Report 2nd Edition, Government Office for Sciences, 2007.

5 Ruppel-Shell E, The Hungry Gene: the science of fat and the future of thin, Atlantic Books, 2003.

6 Foxcroft L, *Calories and Corsets: A history of dieting over 2,000 years*, Profile Books, 2011.

7 Banting W, *Letter on Corpulence*, Fourth Edition, published by Harrison, 1869.

8 Atkins R, *Dr Atkins' Diet Revolution*, Bantam Press, 1972.

9 Taubes G, *Good Calories, Bad Calories*, Anchor Books, 2007.

10 *Soft Drink Contracts in Schools*, The Prevention Institute for the Center for Health Improvement, Oakland, California, May 2002.

11 Yang Q, *Gain weight by "going diet" Artificial sweeteners and the neurobiology of sugar cravings*, Yale Journal of Medicine, June 2010; 83(2): 101-8.

12 Cook D, Haslam D, Weir C, *The role of low calorie sweeteners in weight management: evidence and practicalities*, Supplement to Diabetes Digest 2013 12(1).

13 Office of National Statistics, Households and families – Social Trends 41, 2011.

14 Monteiro C, *The big issue is ultra-processing*, Journal of the World Public Health Nutrition Association, Nov 2010:1(6).

15 ibid, 14.

16 ibid, 4.

17 American Academy of Pediatrics (joint authorship), *Cardiovascular risk reduction in high-risk pediatric populations*, Pediatrics, 2007; 119: 618.

18 Bhaskaran K, Douglas I, et al, *Body-mass index and risk of 22 specific cancers: a population study of 5.24 million UK adults*, The Lancet, Aug 2014; Vol 384: 755-65.

19 Wotton C J, Goldacre M J, *Age at obesity and association with subsequent dementia: record linkage study*, Postgraduate Medical Journal, Aug 2014.

20 de las Fuentes L, Waggoner A D, et al. *Effect of moderate diet-induced weight loss and weight regain on cardiovascular*

structure and function, Journal of the American College of Cardiology, Dec 2009; 54(25):2376-81.

21 Fletcher A M, *Thin for Life: 10 keys to success from people who have lost weight and kept it off*, Chapters Publishing Ltd, 1994.

22 National Weight Control Registry, Brown Medical School, University of Colorado, USA. www.nwcr.ws

23 Wing R R, Phelan S, *Long-term weight loss maintenance*, American Journal of Clinical Nutrition, 2005; 82: 2225-55.

24 Thomas J G, Wing R R, *Maintenance of Long-Term Weight Loss*, Feb 2009, Rhode Island Medicine and Health: 92(2).

25 Wing R R, Hill J O, *Successful Weight Loss Maintenance,* Annual Review of Nutrition, 2001; 21:323-41.

26 Wadden T A , Frey D L, *A multicenter evaluation of a proprietary weight loss program for the treatment of marked obesity: A five-year follow-up*, International Journal of Eating Disorders Sept 1997, 22(2):203-12.

27 Anderson J W, Vichitbandra S, et al, *Long-term weight maintenance after an intensive weight-loss program,* Journal of the American College of Nutrition, Dec 1999; 18(6):620-7.

28 McGuire M T, Wing R R, Klem M L, Hill J O, *Behavioural strategies of individuals who have maintained long-term weight loss,* Obesity Research, Jul 1999; 7(4): 334-41.

29 ibid, 25.

30 ibid, 21.

31 ibid, 24.

32 ibid, 25.

33 ibid, 21 & 23.

34 Klem ML, Wing RR , Lang W, et al, *Does weight loss maintenance become easier over time?* Obesity Research, Sep 2000; 8(6): 438-44.

35 Rastmanesh, Gluck, *"Food Offerings": A Major Factor Impeding Adherence with Weight Loss Diets in Overweight and Obese Individuals,* Journal of Nutritional Disorders and Therapy; 2013 3(1).

36 ibid, 24.

37 Ewbank P P, Darga L L, Lucas C P, *Physical activity as a predictor of weight maintenance in previously obese subjects,* Obesity Research , May 1995, 3(3):257-63.

38 Nelson M. E, Rejeski W J, Blair S N, et al, *Physical activity and public health in older adults: Recommendation from the American College of Sports Medicine and the American Heart Association.* Circulation, 2007; 116(9):1094-1105.

39 Bickel C, Bamman M, et al, *Exercise dosing to retain resistance training adaptations in young and older adults,*

Medicine & Science in Sport & Exercise, July 2011;
43(7):1177-87.

40 McGuire M T, Wing R R, et al, *What predicts weight
regain in a group of successful weight losers?* Journal of
Consulting and Clinical Psychology, Apr 1999; 67(2): 177-85.

41 ibid, 23, 35 & 40.

42 ibid, 24.

43 Butryn M L, Phelan S, Hill J O, Wing R R, *Consistent self-
monitoring of weight: a key component of successful weight
loss maintenance*, Obesity (Silver Spring), Dec 2007;
15(12):3091-6.

44 Elfhag K, Rössner S. *Who succeeds in maintaining weight
loss? A conceptual review of factors associated with weight
loss maintenance and weight regain*, 2005 The International
Association for the Study of Obesity. Obesity reviews 6 , 67–85.

45 ibid, 34.

46 ibid, 21.

47 Niemeier H M, Phelan S, et al, *Internal Disinhibition
Predicts Weight Regain Following Weight Loss and Weight
Loss Maintenance,* Obesity (Silver Spring), Oct
2007;15(10):2485-94.

48 Miller, W R, C'de Baca, J, *Quantum Change: When
Epiphanies and Sudden Insights Transform Ordinary Lives,*
Guilford Publications (Kindle Edition), Oct 2011.

49 National Weight Control Registry, Brown Medical School, University of Colorado, USA. www.nwcr.ws

50 Gorin A A, Phelan S, Hill J O, Wing R R, *Medical triggers are associated with better short- and long-term weight loss outcomes*, Preventive Medicine 39 (2004) 612– 616.

51 ibid, 50.

52 Wing R R, Phelan S, *Long-term weight loss maintenance*, American Journal of Clinical Nutrition, 2005; 82: 2225-55.

53 ibid, 50.

54 ibid, 21.

55 Ballard, Elise, *Epiphany: True Stories of Sudden Insight to Inspire, Encourage, and Transform*, Crown Publishing Group (Kindle Edition), 2011.

56 ibid, 48.

57 Forcehimes A A, *De Profundis : Spiritual Transformations in Alcoholics Anonymous* JCLP/In Session, Vol. 60(5), 503– 517 (2004).

58 ibid, 21.

59 Office of National Statistics, Households and families – Social Trends 41, 2011.

60 Rastmanesh, Gluck, *"Food Offerings": A Major Factor Impeding Adherence with Weight Loss Diets in Overweight and Obese Individuals,* Journal of Nutritional Disorders and Therapy; 2013 3(1).

61 Fritz R, *The Path of Least Resistance*, Newfane Press, electronic publishing, 2010.

62 ibid, 61.

63 Keys A., Brozek J., Henschel A., Mickelsen, O., Taylor, H.L., *The Biology of Human Starvation*, Vol 1-2, University of Minnesota Press, 1950.

64 Benedict F.G., *Human Vitality and Efficiency under Prolonged Restricted Diet*, published by the Carnegie Institution of Washington, 1919. (available online at www.openlibrary.org).

65 Kalm L M, Semba R D, *They Starved so that Others be Better Fed: Remembering Ancel Keys and the Minnesota Experiment*, The Journal of Nutrition, vol 135:1347-52, 2005.

66 ibid, 66.

67 Dulloo A G, Jacquet J, Girardier L, *Poststarvation hyperphagia and body fat overshooting in humans: a role for feedback signals from lean and fat tissues*, The American Journal of Clinical Nutrition, 65:717-23, 1997.